Peter Otto · Klaus Ewe

Atlas of Rectoscopy and Colonoscopy

Translated by B. Clowdus

With 124 Figures in Color (21 Plates)
and 31 Figures Within the Text

Springer-Verlag
Berlin Heidelberg New York 1979

Prof. Dr. P. OTTO
Medizinische Abteilung, Kreiskrankenhaus
3006 Großburgwedel/FRG

Prof. Dr. K. EWE
I. Med. Klinik und Poliklinik der Universität Mainz,
Langenbeckstraße 1, 6500 Mainz/FRG

Translator:
Prof. Dr. B. CLOWDUS, F.A.C.P.
Am Winterberg 2, 3400 Göttingen/FRG

Cover picture: Figures 1–4 of Plate XIII, p. 95

Translation of the 2nd German Edition 1977

ISBN-13: 978-3-642-67252-1 e-ISBN-13: 978-3-642-67250-7
DOI: 10.1007/978-3-642-67250-7

Library of Congress Cataloging in Publication Data. Otto, Peter. Atlas of rectoscopy and colonoscopy. Translation of the 2d ed. of Atlas der Rectoskopie und Coloskopie. Includes bibliographies and index.
1. Proctosigmoidoscopy–Atlases. I. Ewe, Klaus, 1931– joint author. II. Title.
RC864.5.08713 616.3'5'0754 79-673

Softcover reprint of the hardcover 1st edition 1979

Reproduction of the figures: Gustav Dreher GmbH, Stuttgart.

Foreword to the First German Edition

Changes in morphology, both macroscopic and microscopic, continue to play a significant role in the diagnosis of colorectal diseases, and their importance has not been lessened by the introduction of more subtile techniques concerned with alterations in biochemistry and immunology. On the contrary, the present level of confidence in morphologic features as the best means for establishing a diagnosis has led to an even wider acceptance of their value. Factors contributing to this development no doubt include the recent technical advances in the field of fiberoptic endoscopy with a cold light source and the availability of better instruments for obtaining mucosal biopsy specimens from the gastrointestinal tract. Proctoscopy with more extensive examination using colonoscopy remains one of the most important examinations that can be performed in both the physician's office and the hospital. In the properly prepared patient, this examination in conjunction with the histologic examination of tissue obtained through mucosal punch biopsy will greatly aid in the clarification of the vast majority of causes for signs and symptoms of colorectal diseases.

It is therefore welcome that these authors have undertaken to compile their techniques and findings in the form of an atlas of rectoscopy and colonoscopy. They have not only emphasized the importance of this subject for both teaching and practice but have also given us an exact presentation of their techniques with critical appraisal of their findings.

This work will provide a source of very valuable information for every student desiring to learn proctoscopy and colonoscopy, and for those physicians who are already proficient and regularly perform these examinations, it will offer additional stimulation and knowledge. With so many atlases already available concerning esophagogastroduodenoscopy and laparoscopy, this atlas of proctoscopy and colonoscopy fills a vacuum in the medical literature.

Prof. Dr. H.A. KÜHN

Preface to the Second German Edition

The great interest with which our atlas of rectoscopy and colonoscopy was received demonstrated that sufficient didactic help was lacking for the student desiring to master this subject. Within 1 year of its publication, the first edition was completely sold out.

Since the first edition was published, new and important developments have occurred in Germany. The increasing incidence of colorectal carcinoma has led to the introduction of a mandatory test for occult blood in the stool during the annual examination of every person over 45 years of age. When a positive finding is obtained, sigmoidoscopy must be performed in addition to the usual digital examination. As a result, sigmoidoscopy is being used at present even more extensively by the family physician. Along with these developments, a new short fiberoptic sigmoidoscope that can be easily operated has been developed. It enables even the relatively inexperienced individual to examine the colon up to the splenic flexure. Since 90% of all polyps and carcinomas of the colon arise in the area between the anus and the splenic flexure, this instrument could provide for earlier recognition and removal of many colorectal tumors. The technical details of this new fiberscope are, therefore, presented in this second edition. We are additionally grateful to Springer-Verlag whose accomodation made it possible for a number of the Figures and Plates to be altered with resultant improvement in their didactic value.

New illustrations in this edition include those showing pneumatosis cystoides supplied by Dr. H. SCHALK, Krankenhaus Hochstift, Worms; solitary rectal ulcer supplied by Dr. A. NEIGER; and ischemic colitis supplied by Prof. Dr. P. DEYHLE, Zurich.

In the preparation of this second edition, the authors have been helped by many kind suggestions from their colleagues, and for this assistance they are most grateful.

Summer 1977 P. OTTO K. EWE

Preface to the First German Edition

Sigmoidoscopy represents the most extensively used endoscopic examination and is performed by a variety of specialists – internists, surgeons, dermatologists, urologists, gynecologists, pediatricians, and general practitioners.

Most of our colleagues have nevertheless been forced to acquire their knowledge about sigmoidoscopy through their own efforts and to evaluate their results without the benefit of outside help. It is particularly for the members of this group that this atlas of rectoscopy and colonoscopy is intended.

Since sigmoidoscopy should always be performed in conjunction with the medical history and inspection of the anal region and be preceded by the digital rectal examination, these aspects have also been considered. As the use of endoscopy to examine those areas of the large bowel above the reach of the proctoscope has become quite common, a chapter devoted to colonoscopy has also been included.

Until recently, there was no current German-language publication that concerned itself extensively with proctology. Then, *Proctology in the Physician's Office* was published by Roschke containing a report of his extensive personal experiences. This work was soon followed by the exceptionally concise and compact *Atlas of Practical Proctology* by Neiger. Both of these publications are devoted primarily to the practice of proctology, while the *Color Atlas of Endoscopy and Biopsy of the Intestinal Tract* by Beck and others largely foregoes any attention to technical details and proctology.

The authors hope that this atlas will be of practical benefit to colleagues endeavoring to become proficient on their own in proctoscopy and also to those with limited experience who might have difficulty making a diagnosis while performing proctoscopy sporadically. The authors' own recollection of such a situation resulted in their preparation of this atlas. Many colleagues have inspired us to work on this atlas. To each of them we express our thanks. Especially deserving of our gratitude are Mrs. A. Werner and Mrs. W. Opel for their help with the illustrations, as well as Dr. K.A. Schulz, Dermatology Clinic Linden/Hannover for the illustrations of the perianal eczema and braod condylomata. The manuscript was kindly prepared by Mrs. B. Kirchniawy in her spare time. We are also grateful to the staff of Springer-Verlag for advice and help during the production of this book.

P. Otto K. Ewe

Contents

1 Introduction

The first portion of this work is devoted to a consideration of the practical aspects of the proctoscopic examination and thus presents the indications for performing a proctologic evaluation, the information that may be obtained from the patient's medical history, an example of a preprinted data form for use in the recording of the physician's findings, the preparation and positioning of the patient, and the preliminary examination of the anus including the digital rectal examination.

The instruments needed to perform proctoscopy are uncomplicated, and the basic tools are inexpensive. The instruments currently available do not really differ from each other except in minor details. In the text, therefore, we have only described the prototype instruments, and details about the proposed advantages of any particular instrument can be obtained from its manufacturer. The concluding portion of the text describes how the proctoscopic and colonoscopic examinations are performed.

The atlas itself is a topographical stratification of the various diseases that may involve the perianal region, the anus, and the adjacent portions of the large bowel as well as their classification according to morphologic criteria, for example, inflammatory bowel diseases and tumors. Since many pathologic findings in the rectum and sigmoid colon are comparable to those in the upper portions of the large bowel, a duplication of these proctoscopic and colonoscopic illustrations has been avoided.

2 Indications for Performing a Proctologic Examination and Endoscopy

Complaints from the patient about discomfort in the anal region, rectal bleeding, and change in bowel habits – especially recent occurrence of constipation or diarrhea or a change in either symptom – as well as tenesmus are obligatory reasons for conducting a proctologic examination. These symptoms should never be ignored or treated by prescription of hemorrhoid suppositories, antispasmodics, analgesics, or laxatives.

Due to the large number of patients with proctologic symptoms who come to see the physician, it may not always be possible for a complete evaluation to be done in every patient (inspection, digital rectal examination, proctoscopy, colonoscopy). In the selection of those examinations that should be performed in any individual patient, the physician may be required to make compromises.

Inspection, Digital Rectal Examination, and Stool Test for Blood

Inspection and digital rectal examination can be sufficient under the following conditions:

1. Absence of positive historical and physical findings and a negative test for blood in the stool (Hemoccult Test, Röhm Pharma, Darmstadt, Germany; Smith, Kline Diagnostics, Philadelphia, United States; Eaton Laboratories Woking Surrey, United Kingdom)
2. Scratching or wetness in the anal area

Proctoscopy, Sigmoidoscopy

Proctosigmoidoscopy is necessary with:

1. a) Grossly visible bleeding from the anus. Bright red bleeding is usually caused by conditions in the lower large bowel and stems frequently from hemorrhoids, but such bleeding can also arise from a polyp or cancer within this region
   b) Positive test for blood in the stool
2. Change in the patient's bowel habits such as recent diarrhea or constipation; involuntary seapage of stool
3. Appearance of knots around the anal sphincter, prolapsing knots or tumors in association with defecation
4. Pencil-sized stools due to a lesion in the anal area or also a stenosing process in the rectum (carcinoma, etc.).

Radiologic evaluation of the rectum is usually difficult and thus does not customarily result in as concise an examination as proctoscopy. A proctoscopic examination should precede the radiologic examination but radiology may contribute to the understanding of findings insufficiently defined by proctoscopy such as stenoses etc.

Sigmoido-Colonoscopy

In comparison to proctoscopy, the performance of this examination is considerably more complicated technically. The handling of the instrument is more difficult, the examination is more time-consuming, and more personnel is required. A clear and concise indication, therefore, should exist before sigmoido-colonoscopy is performed.

Indications for sigmoido-colonoscopy include:

1. Proctoscopy has not revealed the cause for a stenosing lesion in the rectosigmoid region
2. The radiologic findings are not specific, especially in cases of diverticulitis associated with carcinoma, polyps or different forms of inflammatory bowel disease
3. A discrepancy exists between the clinical history and the negative radiologic findings, or the X-ray and proctoscopic examinations have not explained recurrent gross bleeding from the large bowel
4. The stool test for occult blood is positive, but the X-ray and proctoscopic examinations are negative
5. Preoperative histologic confirmation of a positive radiologic finding

6. Case observation and postoperative evaluation of the therapeutic result as with precancerous lesions, colon resection with anastomosis, removal of colon polyps showing focal carcinoma, or frank malignancy
7. Operative colonoscopy –
   Now that the relatively easy-to-handle "short" fiberoptic sigmoidoscope is available, the indications for sigmoido-colonoscopy have been considerably broadened and approach those for proctoscopy

Contraindication for sigmoido-colonoscopy are:

1. Grossly uncooperative patient
2. Acute inflammatory bowel disease (fulminant ulcerative colitis, toxic megacolon, acute diverticulitis)
3. Acute peritonitis
4. Care should be taken with patients who suffer from coronary heart disease and pulmonary insufficiency.

References

Bohlmann, F.W., Katon, R.M., Lipschutz, G.R., McCool, M.F., Smith, F.W., Melnyk, C.S.: Fiberoptic pansigmoidoscopy. An evaluation and comparison with rigid sigmoidoscopy. Gastroenterology *72*, 644 (1977)

Christie, J.P., Shinya, H.: Indications for fiberoptic colonscopy. South. Med. J. *68*, 881 (1975)

Dean, F.M.: Carcinoma of the colon and rectum – A perspective of practicing physicians with recommendations for screening. West. J. Med. *126*, 431 (1977)

Demling, L., Classen, M., Frühmorgen, P.: Atlas der Enteroskopie. Heidelberg, New York: Springer 1974

Gilbertsen, V.A.: Proctosigmoidoscopy and polypectomy in reducing the incidence of rectal cancer. Cancer *34* [Suppl.], 936 (1974)

Neiger, A.: Atlas der praktischen Proktologie. Bern, Stuttgart, Wien: Huber 1973

Otto, P.: Die ambulante Sigmoidoskopie. Indikation, Technik und Ergebnisse. In: Ergebnisse der Angiologie. Vol. 2.6, Gummrich, H., Nikolowski, W. (eds.). Stuttgart, New York: Schattauer 1973

Otto, P., Bunnemann, H.: Erste Erfahrungen bei der klinischen Abklärung positiver Haemoccult-Tests im Rahmen der neuen kolorektalen Krebsvorsorge im ersten Halbjahr 1977. In: Early detection of colorectal cancer. Goerttler, Kl. (ed.). Nürnberg: Wachholz 1978

Powers, J.H.: Proctosigmoidoscopy in private practice. J. Am. Med. Assoc. *231*, 750 (1975)

Roschke, W.: Die proktologische Sprechstunde, 4th ed. Munich, Berlin, Vienna: Urban & Schwarzenberg 1976

Weiss, W., Hanak, H., Huber, A.: Effizienz der rektal-digitalen Untersuchung zur Früherkennung des Dickdarmkarzinoms. Wien. Klin. Wochenschr. *89*, 654 (1977)

Williams, C.B., Hunt, R.H., Loose, H., Riddell, R.H., Sakai, Y., Swarbrick, E.T.: Colonoscopy in the management of colon polyps. Br. J. Surg. *61*, 673 (1974)

Winawer, S.J., Sherlock, P.: Detecting early colon cancer. Hosp. Pract. *12*, 49 (1977)

3 Clinical History

In the vast majority of cases, a carefully obtained medical history will contribute significantly to the establishment of the diagnosis since most of the symptoms of proctologic diseases are typical. In the following table, the patient's symptoms are compared with their possible cause.

Proctologic history and findings

1. Rectal bleeding	
Blood drops	Perianal thrombosis (spontaneously opened), hemorrhoids
Bright red blood on stool or toilet tissue	Anal fissure, perianal thrombosis (spontaneously opened), hemorrhoids, low lying rectal carcinoma or polyp
Tarry stool	As a rule, bleeding from the upper gastrointestinal tract but also from the colon
Mixed with stool and/or mucus	Ulcerative colitis (rarely Crohn's disease), infectious colitis, radiation colitis, ischemic colitis, carcinoma or polyp
Associated with menstruation	Rectal endometriosis
2. Pain	
Sudden pain in association with defecation, severe, burning, epicritic	Acute fissure in ano
Intermittent or following defecation, dull, burning, terebrant	Incomplete fistula in ano, cryptitis, papillitis
Constant pain	Perianal thrombosis, periproctitial abscess, anal fistula
Cramping	Proctalgia fugax (cramping of the pelvic floor)
Pressing, possibly occurring with defecation	Proctocolitis of various origins, spasm with irritable colon
Sensation of foreign body and/or heavy feeling	Hemorrhoids, especially with prolapse, anal polyps, anal fibroma or advanced anal carcinoma
3. Defecation	
Diarrhea	Functional, colica mucosa ("mucus colitis") irritable colon, colitis, diverticulitis, carcinoma (alternating with constipation)

Constipation	Functional, "habitual constipation," Hirschsprung's disease, carcinoma (alternating with diarrhea)
"Proctogenic constipation"	Fissure, hemorrhoids, anal prolapse, etc.
Pencil-sized stools or notched stools	Lesions located in the anorectal area (for example, carcinoma, hypertrophied anal papilla, polyps), spasm of the anal sphincter (anal fissure, scarring)
Mucus, mucus mixed with stool, passage of "membranes"	Colica mucosa ("mucus colitis") mucosal irritation from other causes
4. Knots in the anal region	
Soft, small skin flaps or folds that do not fill up during abdominal pressing	Hemorrhoidal tags (residua after fissures, perianal thrombosis, overstretching of the anal skin)
Soft knots covered by outside skin that fill up during abdominal pressing	External hemorrhoids (rare)
"Infiltrated" skin folds, "edematous plug," mostly at posterior commissure	"Sentinel fold," the distal end of an anal fissure
Livid, suddenly appearing, tautly elastic, painful knot	Acute perianal thrombosis
Wart-like, sand-colored, small knots arranged like blades of grass	Condylomata acuminata (virus origin), condylomata lata (lues)
Hard, often ulcerating excrescence	Anal carcinoma (rare)
Prolapsing knots	
Whitish, yellowish, hard knots	Hypertrophic anal papillae, fibroma
Bright red knots, up to a child's head in size, convoluted appearance (rectal mucosa)	Anal-rectal prolapse
Pea- to plum-sized knot(s) covered with mucous membrane, partly fibrosed	Hemorrhoids, grade II and III (secondary anal prolapse)
5. Pruritus ani	Often no pathological findings visible, anal eczema, acute-chronic, hemorrhoids, infestation with worms

Name and address of clinic	Name and address of patient

Proctologic examination

Reason for consultation:
Complaints:

Pain
Wetness
Itching
Bleeding: mixed with stool
separate from stool
Mucus discharge

Bowel movement
Laxatives
Anal operation
Other:

Inspection:

Redness, eczema
Hemorrhoid tags
Fissure
Hemorrhoids
Fistula
Prolapse
Perianal thrombosis

dorsal

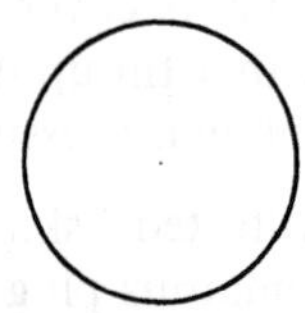

ventral

Digital examination:

Sphincter tone
Scarring, stenosis
Tumor, resistance
Prostate
Cervix

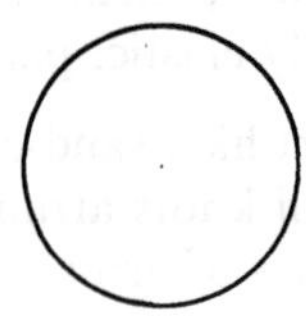

Proctoscopy:

Hemorrhoids – grade I...... II......
Hypertrophied papillae
Tumor

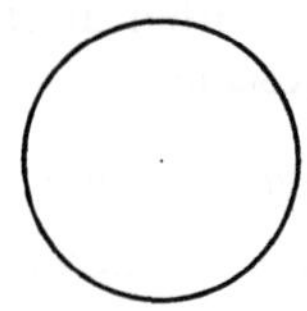

Proctosigmoidoscopy: to cm......

Spasm
Mucosa
Vascularity
Tumor
Other findings
Photo at cm:
Biopsy at cm:

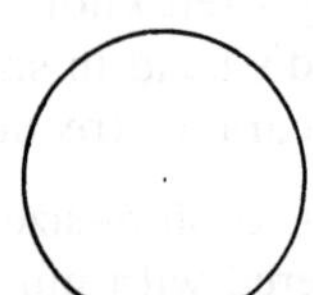

Diagnosis:

Return visit on: ....

Treatment:

(Signature)

3.1 Preprinted Record Form

The form shown on page 6 is useful for recording clinical findings and recommended therapy.

References

Buie, L.A.: Practical proctology, 2nd ed. Springfield (Ill.): C.C. Thomas 1960
Cook, G.B.: A form for recording proctosigmoidoscopic examinations. Am. J. Surg. *133*, 264 (1977)
Neiger, A.: Atlas der praktischen Proktologie. Bern, Stuttgart, Vienna: Huber 1973
Roschke, W.: Die proktologische Sprechstunde, 4th ed. Munich, Berlin, Vienna: Urban & Schwarzenberg 1976
Williams, J.F., Thomson, J.P.: Ano-rectal bleeding: A study of causes and investigative yields. Practitioner *219*, 327 (1977)

4 Preparation for Endoscopic Examination

Inspection of the perianal area, the digital rectal examination, and the proctoscopic examination may be done without special preparation.

4.1 Proctosigmoidoscopy

For preparation before proctosigmoidoscopy, a Fleet enema is recommended. This usually results in cleaning the colon up to the splenic flexure.

In the acute phase of ulcerative colitis, the characteristic features of the disease (purulent-bloody lining) are better recognized without any preparation. Prior preparation with laxatives, special diets, or high enemas is not required. The patient evacuates the enema within 10–20 min, and the examination should be performed within 15–20 min thereafter before the bowel contents from above enter the cleansed portion of the colon.

4.2 Sigmoidocolonoscopy

In preparation for sigmoidocolonoscopy, it is necessary to distinguish between extended sigmoidoscopy to the splenic flexure ("partial" colonoscopy) and actual colonoscopy to the cecum ("total" or "high" colonoscopy).

4.2.1 Extended Sigmoidoscopy

The preparation described under Sect. 4.1 using a Fleet enema is also sufficient here.

4.2.2 High Colonoscopy

For high colonoscopy under clinical conditions, two high enemas using 1,500 ml water containing 5 ml bisacodyl 4 and 1 h before the examination are recommended. The patient should be turned during the administration of the enema from the left side over the stomach to the right side so that the enema can reach the cecum. Approximately 30 min before the actual examination, an additional Fleet enema is given to remove any residual colon contents in the ampulla.

For thorough cleansing of the colon recently "Saline lavage" has been recommended by Levy et al. The patient has to drink $^3/_4$ l of an isotonic electrolyte solution (see below) hourly up to a maximum of 6 l until the fluid which is discharged from the rectum is relatively clear and free of particulate matter. Isotonic manitol solution can be given instead which is to be tolerated better by the patient.

NaCl 6.5 g
$NaHCO_3$ 2.5 g
KCl 0.75 g
aqua dest ad 1000.0

The expensive "astronaut elemental" diets often leave behind a dark, sticky coating on the mucosa that is difficult to remove with enemas and can be mistaken for a tarry stool.

For preparation of outpatients, we recommend that the patient be given a daily dose of bisacodyl at 1400 h on the 2 days prior to the colonoscopic examination, as well as a liquid or low-residue diet on the day before the examination. In the early morning of the day of the examination, the patient should be given a Fleet enema.

4.3 Endoscopic Polypectomy

When a polyp is to be removed from the distal colon (descending and sigmoid) – the most common location for colon polyps – the preparation described under Sect. 4.1 for sigmoidoscopy should be used since complications requiring corrective surgery following the endoscopic removal of polyps have rarely been described.

4.4 Premedication for Sigmoidocolonoscopy

Analgesics and spasmolytic agents make the introduction of the instrument more difficult and painful because the relaxed bowel tends to become overly distended during introduction of the colonoscope with excessive stretching and loop formation in the sigmoid colon. If sedation is used Valium i.v. is preferable in 5–10 mg dosage.

References

Bohlman, T.W., Katon, R.M., Lipshutz, G.R., McCool, M.F., Smith, F.W., Melnyk, C.S.: Fiberoptic pansigmoidoscopy. An evaluation and comparison with rigid sigmoidoscopy. Gastroenterology *72*, 644 (1977)

Demling, L., Classen, M., Frühmorgen, P.: Atlas der Enteroskopie. Berlin, Heidelberg, New York: Springer 1974

Deyhle, P.: Fiberoptic colonoscopy. In: Gastroenterology, 3r ed. Bockus, H.L. (ed.), Vol. II. Philadelphia: Saunders 1976

Evans, K.: The use of bisacodyl suppositories in preparation for sigmoidoscopy. Gut 5, 172 (1964)
Levy, A.G., Benson, J.W., Hewlett, E.L., Hardt, J.R., Doppman, J.L., Gordon, R.S. Jr.: Saline lavage: A rapid, effective and acceptable method for cleansing the gastrointestinal tract. Gastroenterology *70*, 157 (1976)
Marino, A.W.J.: Types of flexible sigmoidoscopes and preparation of the patient. Dis. Colon Rectum *20*, 91 (1977)
Otto, P., Huchzermeyer, H., Müller, H.: Komplikationen bei der Coloskopie – Ergebnis einer Umfrage an gastroenterologischen Zentren in der Bundesrepublik Deutschland. In: Fortschritte in der Endoskopie. Kongreßbericht des 9. Kongresses der Deutschen Gesellschaft für Endoskopie. Munich 1976. Erlangen: peri med 1976
Smith, L.E., Nivatvongs, S.: Complications in colonoscopy. Dis. Colon Rectum *18*, 214 (1975)
Williams, C.B., Hunt, R.H., Loose, H., Riddell, R.H., Sakai, Y., Swarbrick, E.T.: Colonoscopy in the management of colon polyps. Br. J. Surg. *61*, 673 (1974)

5 Position

Three positions are recommended for proctoscopy: (1) the knee-elbow position, (2) the dorsal lithotomy position, and (3) Sims's position. The optimal proctoscopic examination depends less on the position of the patient and more on the skill and experience of the examiner – each position has its advantages and disadvantages.

5.1 Knee-Elbow or Knee-Chest Position (Fig. 1a and 1b)

Advantages. Good visualization of the perianal region with optimal conditions for proctosigmoidoscopy – the abdominal contents fall cephalad and the sigmoid colon stretches. Insufflation of air is usually unnecessary.

Disadvantages. The position is relatively uncomfortable for most patients; for ill and elderly individuals it is less acceptable and for examinations of long duration it is less appropriate.

Performance of the examination. The patient kneels on a high table (operating, endoscopy, or examining table) as close as possible to the examiner and by leaning forward either bears his weight on his elbows or on his chest (Fig. 1a)

It is much easier for the patient to assume this position if a special tilting proctoscope table is used (Fig. 1b and 1c; see also Fig. 11). This table can also be used for the dorsal lithotomy position by attaching leg supports (Fig. 1c).

5.2 Dorsal Lithotomy Position (Fig. 1c)

Advantages. A gynecologic examining table is almost always present in most physicians' offices and clinics. This position is not only favorable for proctoscopic examination but is also more comfortable for the patient than the knee-elbow position.

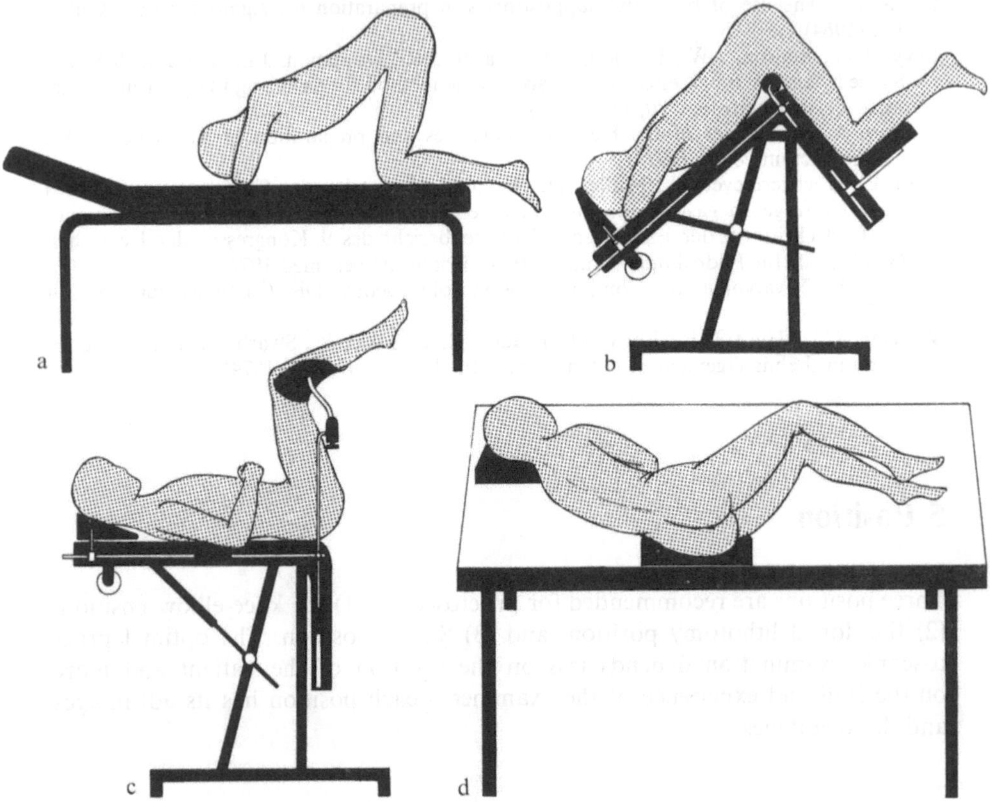

Fig. 1a–d. Positioning for proctoscopy. **a** knee-elbow position; possible with any table; **b** knee-elbow or knee-chest position using the tiltable proctoscopic table after Ewe; **c** dorsal lithotomy position; **d** Sims's position.

Disadvantage. The abdominal contents lie on top of the sigmoid colon and compromise the lumen of the bowel. To maintain an open lumen, air must be repeatedly insufflated.

5.3. Sims's Position (Fig. 1d)

This position is seldom used in Germany but is rather common in the United Kingdom.

Advantages. The position is comfortable for the patient. In emergency situations and with very ill patients, the examination can also be performed in bed. Proctoscopy can be easily done, and the sigmoid colon also stretches. Insufflation of air is, however, necessary in most patients. This position includes characteristics of the other two positions.

Disadvantage. In comparison to the other two positions, the examiner's freedom of motion is rather limited.

Performance of the Examination. The patient lies on a high examination table on his left side with his buttocks supported by a pillow.

References

Buie, L.A.: Practical proctology, 2nd ed. Springfield (Ill.): C.C. Thomas 1960
Haubrich, W.S.: Proctosigmoidoscopy. In: Gastroenterology, 3rd ed. Bockus, H.L. (ed.), Vol. II. Philadelphia: Saunders 1976
Jackman, R.J.: Rigide tube proctosigmoidoscopy. In: Gastrointestinal panendoscopy. Berry, L.H. (ed.). Springfield (Ill.): C.C. Thomas 1974
Neiger, A.: Atlas der praktischen Proktologie. Bern, Stuttgart, Vienna: Huber 1973
Nesselrod, J.P.: Clinical proctology. Philadelphia, London: Saunders 1957
Roschke, W.: Die proktologische Sprechstunde, 4th ed. Munich, Berlin, Vienna: Urban & Schwarzenberg 1976

6 Inspection of the Perianal Region

During inspection of the perianal region and the anus, a portion of the anal canal may also be examined through stretching of the buttocks (Fig. 13). Good illumination is needed for an optimal examination.

Important findings that may be obtained through inspection (see also Sect. 12) are:

acute and chronic eczema, fistulous tract openings, perirectal abscess, condylomata, skin tags, perianal thrombosis (hematoma), external hemorrhoids, prolapsing internal hemorrhoids (grade III), anal and rectal prolaps, anal carcinoma, tears, fissures, and "sentinel folds".

The patient is then requested to "bear down," which makes it possible for the examiner to gain further information about expanding *external* or *prolapsing internal hemorrhoids (grade II), anal and rectal prolapse, or hypertrophied anal papillae.*

7 Digital Rectal Examination (Fig. 2a and 2b)

7.1 Finger Protection

During examination of the anal region and before doing the rectal examination, the hand is protected by a *plastic glove.* A number of disposable gloves of varying strengths are on the market. One may additionally use a *finger cot* on the forefinger, which is removed after the examination. The examination can also be done using a finger cot alone with the finger stuck through a piece of gauze that protects the rest of the hand. Right-handed examiners often elect to use the forefinger of the left hand for the rectal examination and keep the right hand uncontaminated for handling instruments.

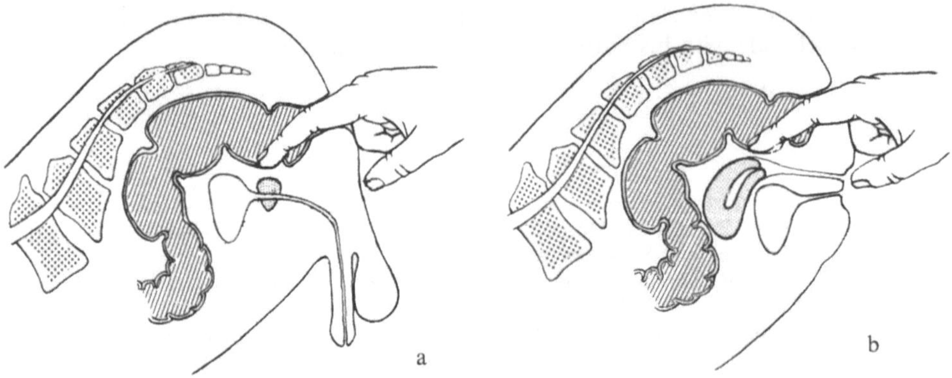

Fig. 2a and b. Schematic presentation of the technique for digital rectal examination. **a** Examination of the male with palpation of the prostate; **b** Examination of the female with palpation of the uterus.

7.2 Practical Performance

The patient must be informed in advance that a finger is to be inserted in to his rectum. He is advised to "bear down" as he does during defecation or to "loosen up completely." The finger has an oval diameter. It is easier on the patient for the finger to be inserted sideways with a rotary downward motion. For a lubricant one may use catheter lubricant, vaseline, or oily salves.

The palpating finger can reach the anus, anal canal (3—5 cm long), and rectum up to approximately 8 cm (Fig. 13). In the dorsal lithotomy position and with bearing down, it may be possible to detect localized resistance beyond this distance. During the examination, the forefinger should make a complete circle. Special attention should be paid to the dorsal proximal area, which cannot be endoscopically visualized. The examiner should note whether any blood is present on his finger after removal. Some patients, especially obese individuals, have a so-called *funnel anus*, in which cases an examination even by an examiner with long fingers is incomplete.

During the examination, attention should be paid to the following:

Pain. Fresh anal fissures are so painful that it may be impossible to perform a digital rectal examination without local anesthesia. *Chronic fissures, tears, cryptitis, papillitis,* and *ulcerations* are painful upon palpation. By applying pressure with the finger in various places, the site may be localized. Pain elicited by pressure on the coccyx is known as "*coccygodynia.*"

Sphincter tone. The tone increases with painful lesions and decreases after operations, as is often the case after difficult deliveries. The competence of the external sphincter can be ascertained by having the patient contract the anal musculature. In the bimanual examination, the sphincter is grasped between the thumb and the examining forefinger, and attention is paid to scarring from fistulae.

Patency. With the digital examination, congenital and acquired stenoses can also be detected. The name "*pectinosis*" is used to describe the condition wherein a fibrous narrowing within the area of the internal sphincter exists, probably the result of a chronic inflammatory process such as anitis, cryptitis, or papillitis.

Resistance. Hemorrhoids are soft, spongy objects that may be pressed out during the examination. As a rule they cannot be felt by the finger. When they are palpable, they are thrombosed or fibrosed or the resistance is due to a new growth (*anal fibroma, hypertrophied anal papilla,* the rare *carcinoma of the anus, postoperative scarring, thrombosed hemorrhoidal knots, polyps, rectal carcinoma*).

Prostate. The following characteristics of the normal prostate are important: *symmetry of the lobes* and *size.* It is not always possible to reach the upper border of the prostate. The normal *consistency* is firm and comparable to the palmar fasciae upon palpation of the hollow of the hand. In cases of carcinoma, a discrete nodule that is as hard as a knuckle may be found, and when the carcinoma is advanced, a whole lobe or the entire prostate may be altered. The displaceability of the mucosa of the prostate upon palpation may be eliminated by carcinomatous infiltration. Extreme pain caused by pressure on the prostate occurs with prostatitis. Hypertrophy of the middle lobe causing urologic symptoms cannot be detected by the digital examination.

Cervix uteri. The cervix may be examined through the rectum. *Gynecologic foreign bodies* such as diaphragms, pessaries, or vaginal tampons may offer firm resistance and confuse the examination findings. Scybala can be misinterpreted as being tumors and can be crushed against the bowel wall.

References

Buie, L.A.: Practical proctology 2nd ed. Springfield (Ill.): C.C. Thomas 1960

Dietrich, K.F.: Proktologie für die Praxis. München: Lehmann 1969

Neiger, A.: Atlas der praktischen Proktologie. Bern, Stuttgart, Vienna: Huber 1973

Nesselrod, J.B.: Clinical proctology Philadelphia, London: Saunders 1957

Roschke, W.: Die proktologische Sprechstunde, 4th ed. Munich, Berlin, Vienna: Urban & Schwarzenberg 1976

8 Instruments Used for Endoscopy of Anus and Rectum*

In the discussion of endoscopic instruments and additional tools, we have referred only to the general features and important principles since instruments from individual firms not only vary in details but are also being continuously modified. The characteristics of any specific instrument may be obtained from its manufacturer.

8.1 Lighting

The modern instruments are illuminated by a fiber-optic *cold light* that has its origin in a light source and is transmitted through the fiber bundles in the endoscope (Fig. 3). The light is attached proximally to the anal specula, anoscope, and rigid rectoscope. With the newer types of proctosigmoidoscopes, the glass fibers run through the outer sheath of the instrument and the light emerges distally 2 cm before the opening (distal lighting, Fig. 5a and 5b). Other brands have the light attached to the proximal portion of the endoscope. Earlier instruments that used bulbs for illumination are no longer appropriate. There are light sources of various strengths on the market. Figure 3 shows the generator 5005 (R. Wolf Medical Instruments Corp. 7046 Lyndon Ave. Rosemont, IL 60018, United States).

8.2 Anal Specula (Fig. 4a and 4b)

The main use for the anal speculum is the documentation of disease processes such as fissures and fistulae in the distal anal canal.

Instruments. One can resort to the use of the vaginal speculum if one is available. Roschke developed a special anal speculum. Additionally, the tripartite speculum developed by the Olympus Corp. to introduce the colonoscope may also be used. The *anal retracter* after Parks is especially useful in small operations in the region of the anal canal or hemorrhoid area.

8.3 Anoscope (Fig. 4c)

The anoscope is particularly useful in evaluating processes within the region of the *linea dentata.* The tip of the instrument is usually beveled. With this instrument *hemorrhoids* can be *injected* (technique of Bensaude, see p. 52).

---

* *Endoscopes and Additional Instruments for Rectoscopy.* The illustrations are limited to the most important prototypes. Further details can be obtained from the various company catalogues (Germany: Richard Wolf GmbH, 7134 Knittlingen; Karl Storz GmbH & Co., 7200 Tuttlingen; United Kingdom: Down Bros. and Meyer + Phelps Ltd., Church Path, Mitcham, Surrey CR4 3UE; United States: Karl Storz Endoscopy America Ltd., 658 South San Vincente Blvd., Los Angeles, CA 90045; Richard Wolf, Medical Instrument Corp., 7046 Lyndon Ave., Rosemont, IL 60018; American Hospital Supply Co., 1450 Waukegan Road, McGraw Park, IL)

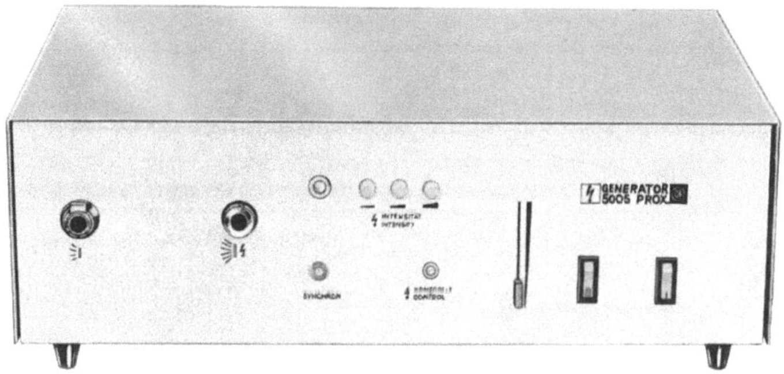

Fig. 3. Light source. The ilumination is obtained from a halogen lamp and is conducted through a fiberoptic bundle to the endoscope (Wolf Co.).

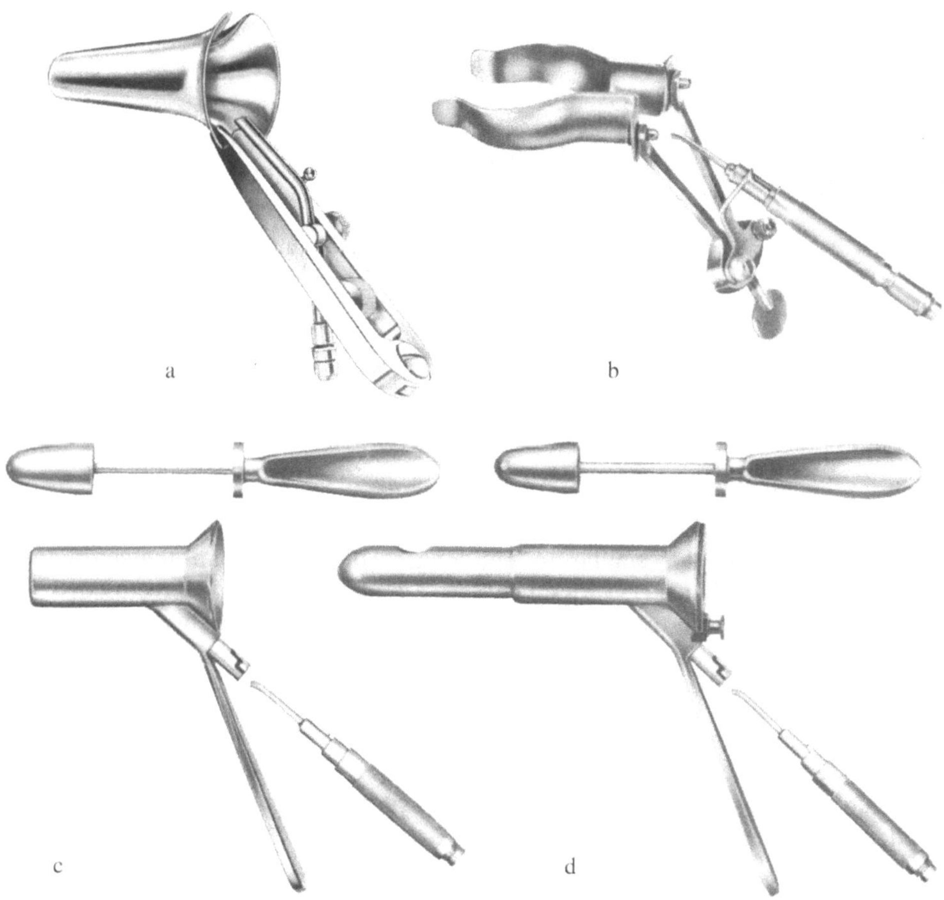

Fig. 4a–d. Endoscopes for the distal portions of the large bowel. **a** anal speculum after Roschke with cold light (Wolf Co.); **b** anal retracter after Parks with cold light (Storz Co.); **c** anoscope (Storz Co.); **d** proctoscope with side window. This model can be inserted through the anoscope.

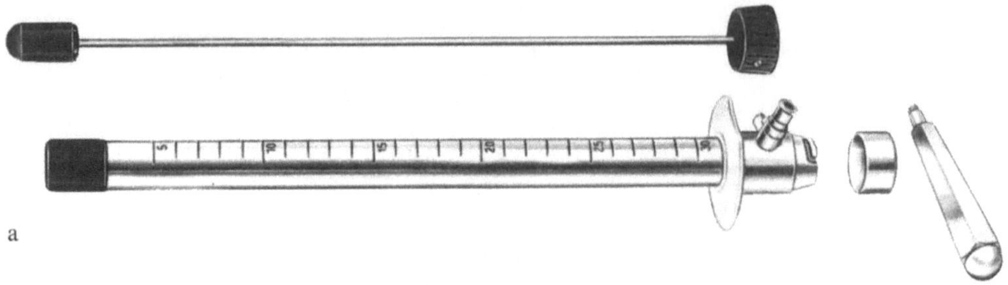

a

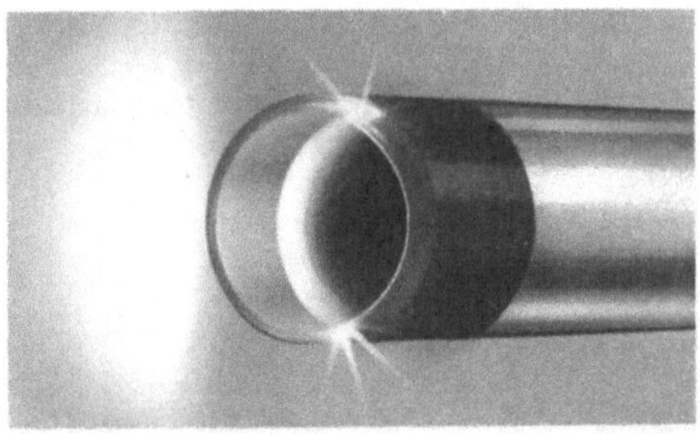

b

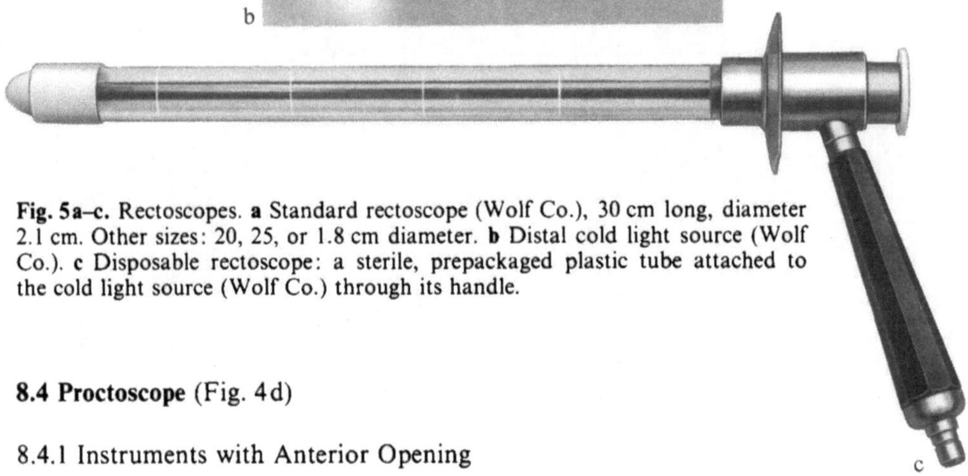

c

Fig. 5a–c. Rectoscopes. **a** Standard rectoscope (Wolf Co.), 30 cm long, diameter 2.1 cm. Other sizes: 20, 25, or 1.8 cm diameter. **b** Distal cold light source (Wolf Co.). **c** Disposable rectoscope: a sterile, prepackaged plastic tube attached to the cold light source (Wolf Co.) through its handle.

8.4 Proctoscope (Fig. 4d)

8.4.1 Instruments with Anterior Opening

These instruments are similar to but longer (10–12 cm) than the anoscope (6–7 cm). Their diameter varies between 1.2 and 2.1 cm. If a rectoscope is present in addition to the anoscope, then a proctoscope is not absolutely necessary.

8.4.2 Instruments with Lateral Opening

Hemorrhoids prolapse into the side openings and are treatable by *injection* after Blond (see p. 51).

8.5 Rectoscope (Fig. 5a–5c)

The standard instrument for rectosigmoidoscopy is 30 cm long and has a diameter of around 2 cm (Fig. 5a). There are also instruments of larger caliber with a diameter of approximately 3 cm (operating rectoscope). The fiber bundles in the instruments from Wolf Co. end distally (Fig. 5b), while those in the Storz instrument end proximally at a head to which the rectoscope tube portion is attached.

Disposable rectoscopes and proctoscopes have recently become available. The plastic tube is connected through its handle to a cold light source (Fig. 5c).

8.6 Pediatric Instruments

Children from the age of 5–6 years can be examined with adult-sized instruments. For infants and younger children, shorter instruments (20 cm) of smaller caliber (1 cm diameter) are available.

a

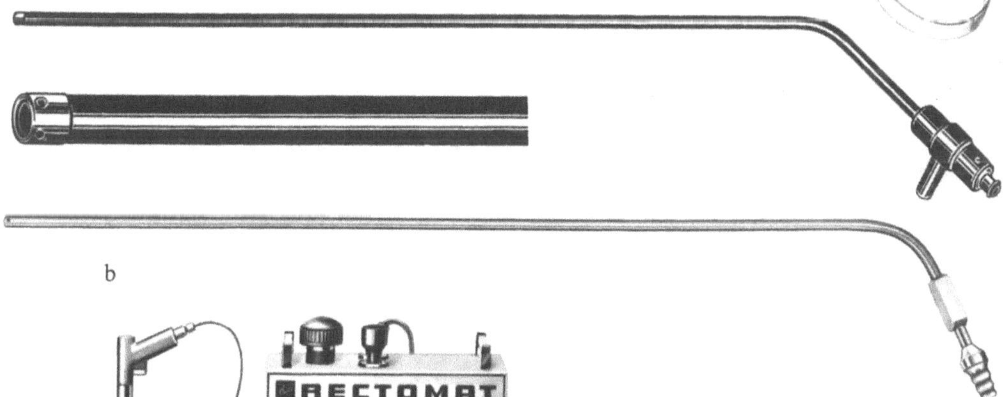

b

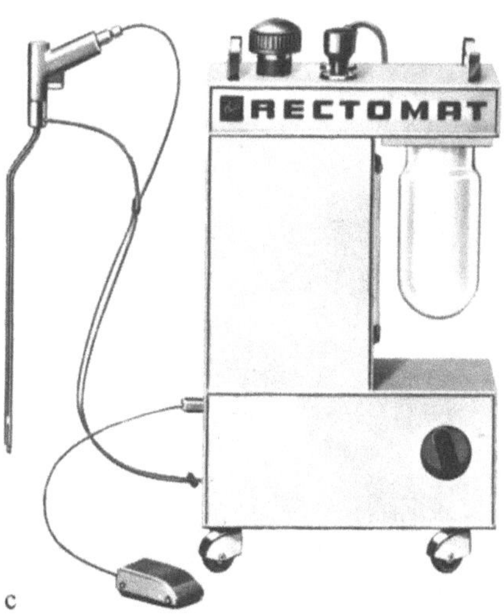

c

Fig. 6a–c. Cleaning Aids. **a** Applicator with three grippers (Wolf Co.). **b** Suction tubes. The insulated suction tube permits simultaneous suction and coagulation. **c** Combination suction and irrigation device "Rectomat" (Liebisch Co., 4812 Brackwede, FRG).

9 Additional Instruments

9.1 Sounds

Button sounds to probe for fistulous tracts as well as sounds with pierced heads for use in placing thread drains are obtainable.

9.2 Cleaning Aids (Fig. 6a–6c)

9.2.1 Applicators

Applicators with forceps, wire baskets, or loops make it possible to grasp and turn cotton swabs and thus to clean the area under examination.

9.2.2 Suction Tubes

Suction tubes are used to remove the remaining enema fluid or liquid stools. They are attached to a conventional suction pump that should have a suction capacity of 600–800 mm Hg. The water faucet pumps are practical and inexpensive.

9.2.3 Suction-Irrigation Devices

Ordinarily, simple suction tubes are adequate to clean the colon of troublesome content. An electronically controlled device exists, however, with which one can irrigate and suction alternately – the transportable *"Rectomat"* (Fa. Liebisch, 4817 Brackwede, FRG).

9.3 Biopsy Instruments (Fig. 7a and 7b)

9.3.1 Forceps

For biopsy sampling of circumscribed lesions (tumors, etc.), various types of biopsy forceps exist; those with a nonconductible shaft also permit electrocoagulation of bleeding areas.

9.3.2 Suction Biopsy

Tissue samples from the mucosa for the use in the determination of various changes may also be obtained using suction biopsy. The complication rate with suction biopsy is lower than with forceps biopsy (Ewe).

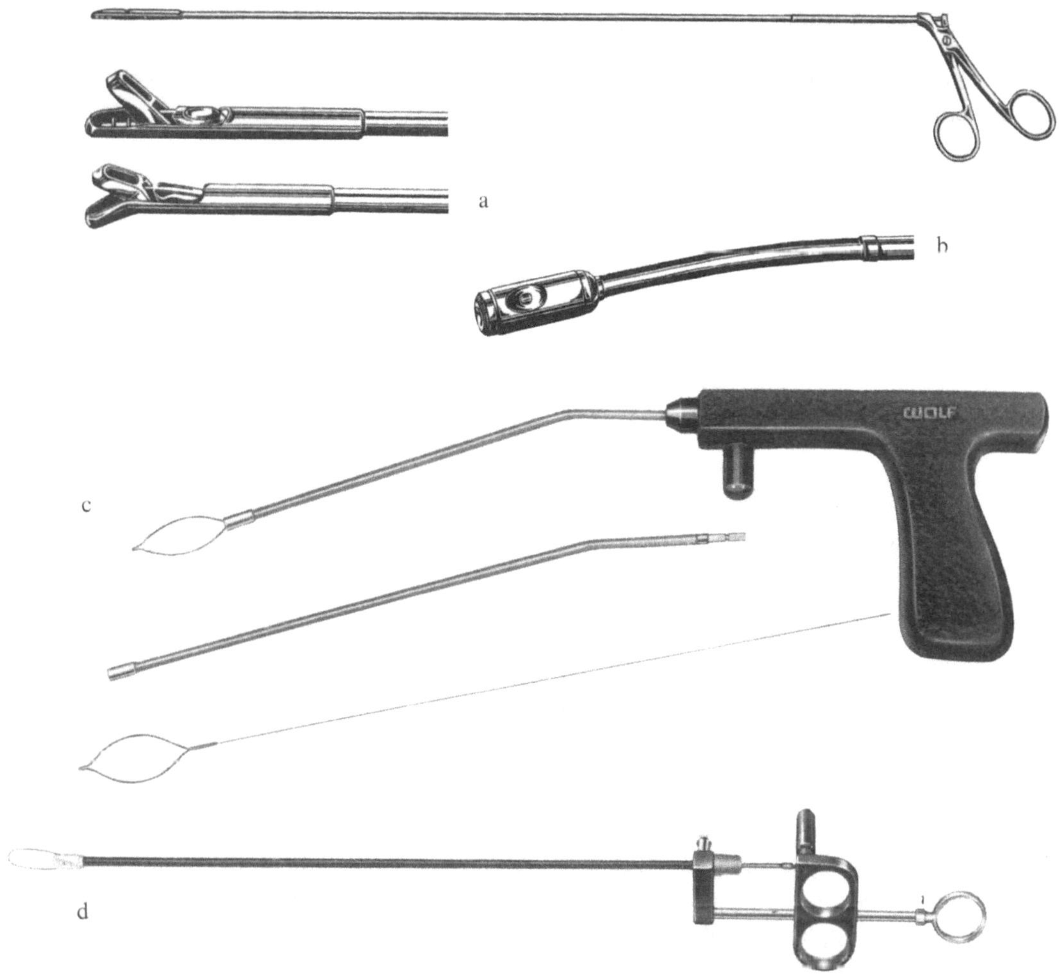

Fig. 7a–d. Biopsy instruments. **a** biopsy forceps with straight and angulated tip; **b** suction biopsy with flexible tip after Ewe (Wolf Co.); **c** polyp snare (Wolf Co.); **d** polyp snare (Storz Co.).

9.4 Polyp Snares (Fig. 7c and 7d)

Polyp snares are wire loops that are connected to a high-frequency device and can be used for cutting coagulation. Still available but not recommended are the wound soft wire loops.

9.5 Coagulation Sounds to Control Bleeding

Especially useful are those coagulation sounds that can simultaneously be used for suction. They permit better definition of the bleeding site and its coagulation.

For electrocoagulation with the polyp snare, one needs a high-frequency generator.

9.6 Curved Knife

For use in the incision of infected crypts (*"cryptotom"*), a curved knife is effective.

9.7 Foreign-Body Forceps

Mobile, long-stemmed polyps can also be fixed for snare excision with foreign-body forceps (Fig. 8).

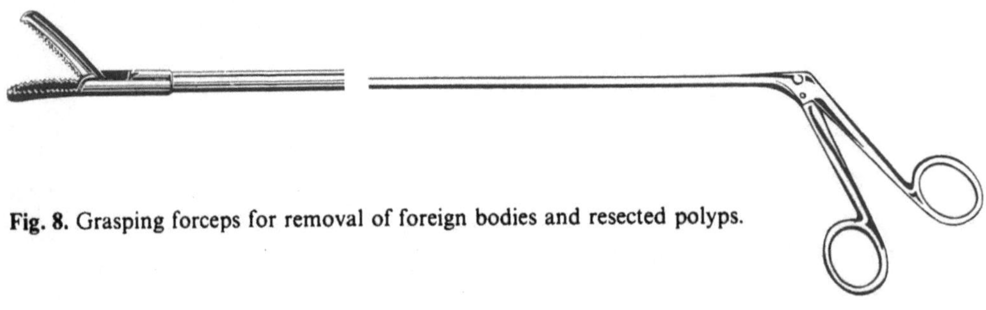

Fig. 8. Grasping forceps for removal of foreign bodies and resected polyps.

9.8 Instruments for Treatment of Hemorrhoids (Fig. 9a–9e)

Injection instruments may be used for sclerosing hemorrhoids. With the Blond method, needles having a straight shaft and a total length of 18 cm are used. The distal tip of the needle is angulated at 45°. Special syringes facilitate the dropwise application of a sclerosing fluid. The needles for use with the Bensaude method are straight throughout their length but have an arresting device to prevent too deep a penetration.

9.9 Optical Aids

9.9.1 Magnifiers (Fig. 10a–10d)

A magnifying glass during endoscopy greatly enhances the perception of details. The magnifying glass is either already attached to the instrument and adjustable (Storz Co.) or it can be attached (telescopic lens, Wolf Co.).

9.9.2 Magnification Attachments (Lumina, Hopkin's Optics)

Even stronger magnification may be obtained with lens systems that can be inserted into the rectoscope. Special types of lens attachments are the Wolf operative device with a bayonet-form, angled optic that enlarges the view of the biopsy area and the Storz optical system using an angled biopsy forceps.

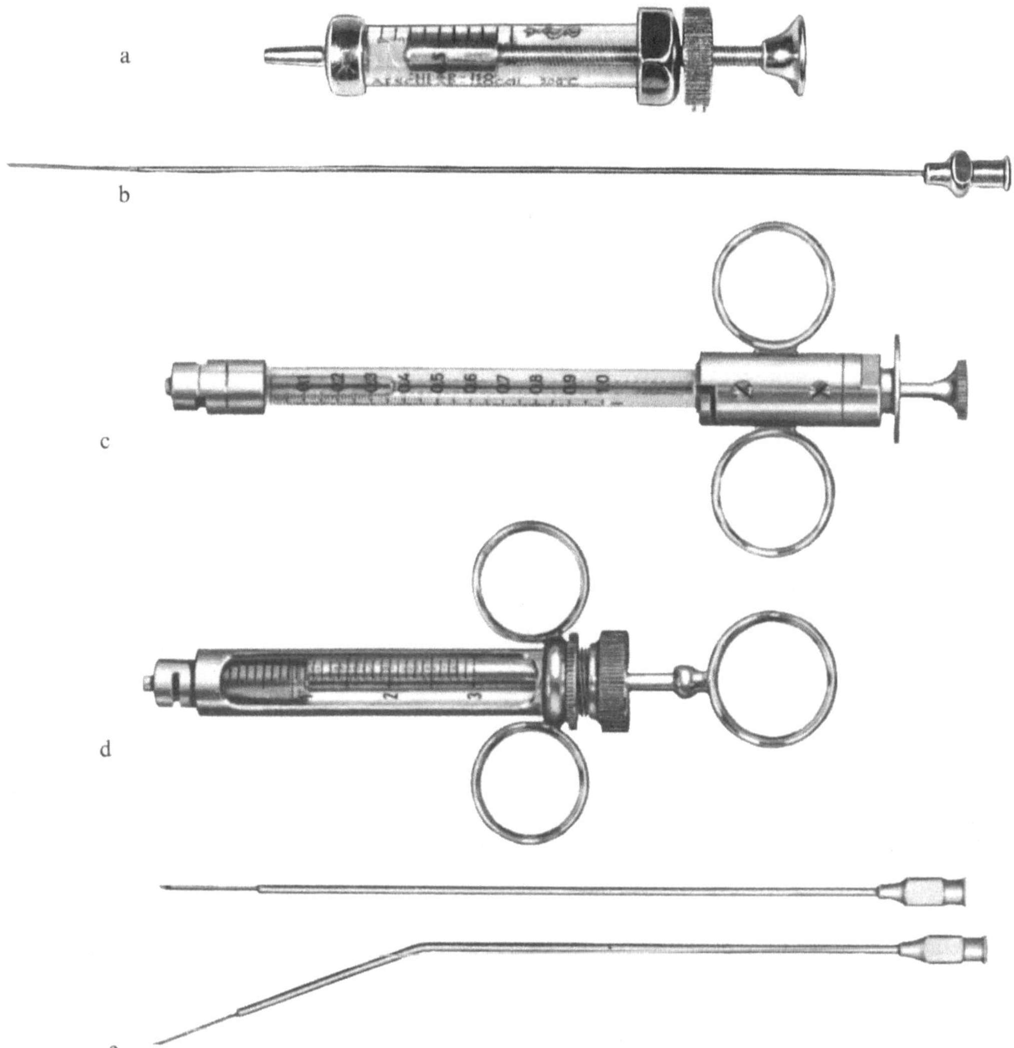

Fig. 9a–c. Hemorrhoid syringes and canulae. **a** drop syringe (1 ml) (Wolf Co.); **b** injection canula with flexible distal portion, 12.5, 15.0, or 20.0 cm long (Wolf Co.); **c** drop syringe after Böhm (1 ml) (Storz Co.); **d** drop syringe after Gabriel (3 ml) (Storz Co.); **e** injection canula with Luer Lock (Storz Co.).

9.10 Documentation by Photography (Fig. 10c)

Electronic flash lighting can be reflected from outside. With the Polaroid camera, it is possible to obtain four color photographs per film that are available within 2 min.

Cameras suitable for endoscopic photography are equipped with special optical systems by the firms making the attachment. A conventional camera may also be modified for use in endoscopic photographic documentation.

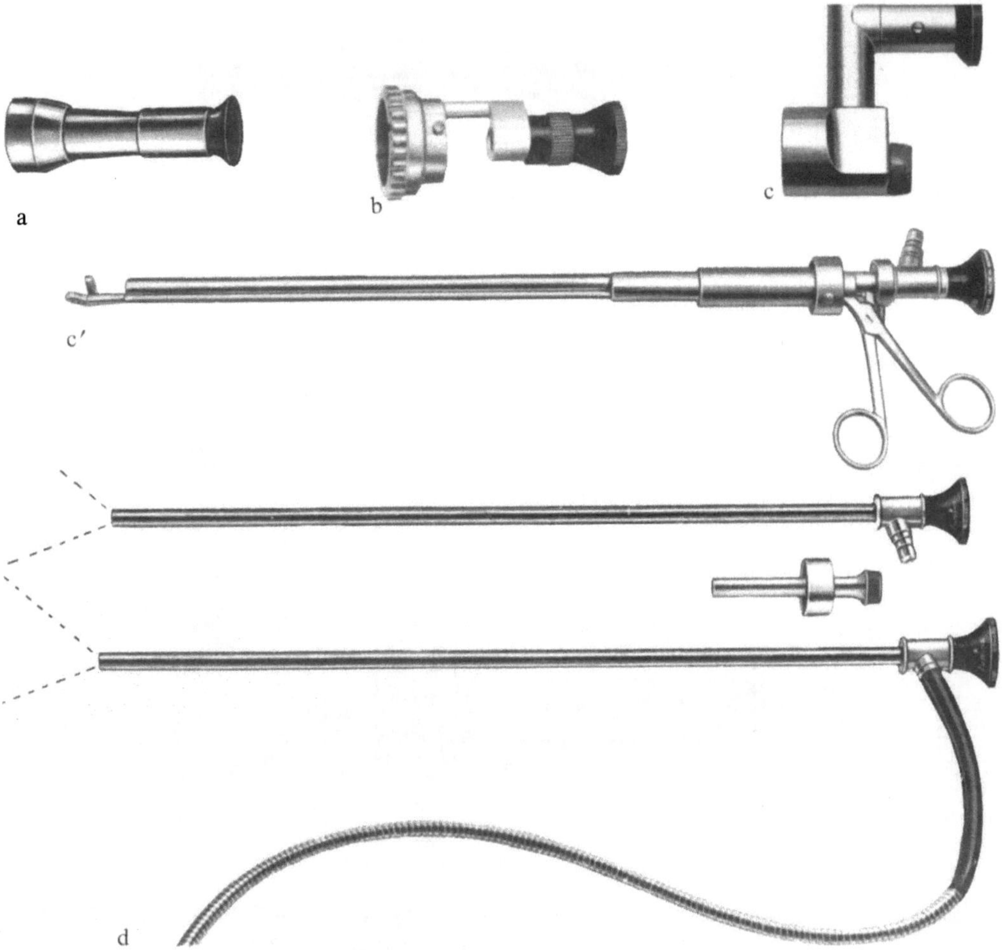

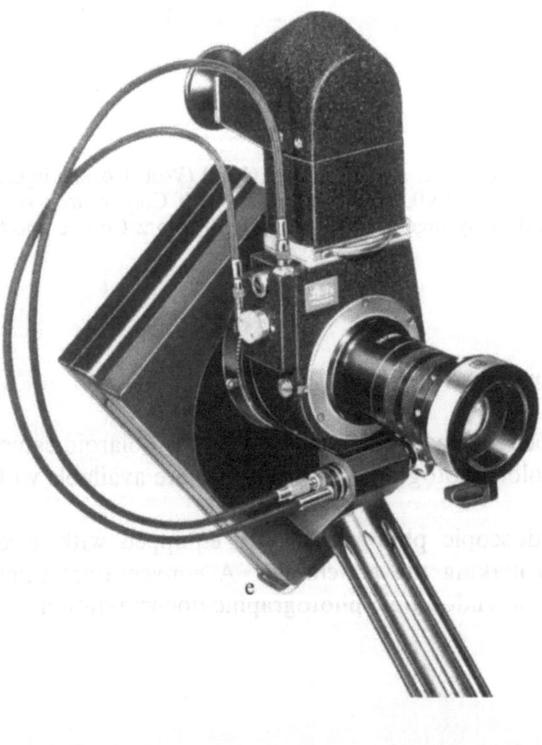

Fig. 10a–e. Optical aids. **a** optical attachment (telescopic lens) (Wolf Co.); **b** adjustable lens (Storz Co.); **c** operation device and optical biopsy forceps (Wolf Co.); **d** lens attachment for magnification during photography; **e** Polaroid camera for rapid documentation of findings (four color pictures).

10 Technique for Performing Rectoscopy

10.1 Introduction of the Instrument (Fig. 13a–d)

After positioning of the patient (Figs. 1 and 11), the instrument is introduced into the anus. The anal canal runs diagonally toward the navel. This distance must be passed blindly. The instrument is therefore guided through this area with the help of the obturator, which is promptly removed after passage of the instrument through the anal canal.

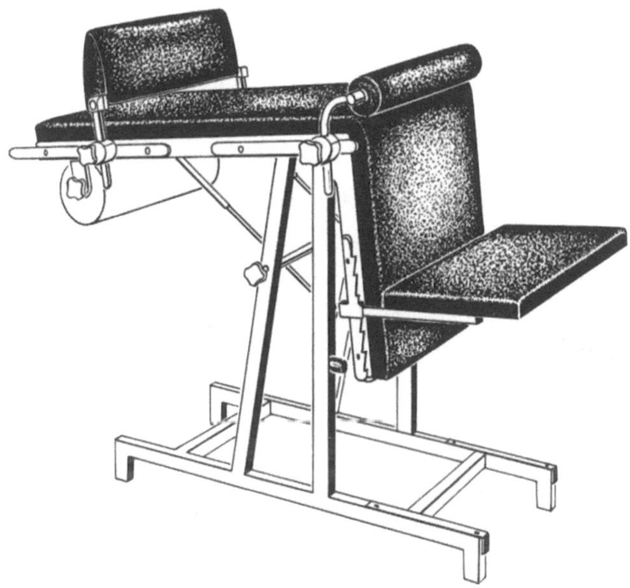

Fig. 11. Rectoscopic examination table after Ewe (Wolf Co.). Can be used for the knee-elbow position as well as the dorsal lithotomy position when leg supports are attached.

10.2 Manipulation of the Instrument During Its Advancement (Fig. 13a–d)

To obtain a complete view of the ampulla, the handle of the rectoscope must be lowered quite considerably in the ventral direction (Fig. 13a). The sigmoid usually begins at a distance of 14–15 cm from the anus. The course of the sigmoid shows marked *individual variation* (Fig. 12a–12d). If the angle is too acute, advancement of the instrument will be impossible even for an expert. If passage through the rectosigmoidal junction causes the patient too much discomfort, the instrument should not be forced. If important indications exist for inspecting this area, a flexible colonoscope can subsequently be used for the examination.

10.3 Normal Findings (Plate I; Fig. 13a–d)

The topography of the anus and the rectosigmoid is depicted in Fig. 14 with information about distances from the external anal sphincter. Various structures can be localized with the centimeter scale of the rectoscope.

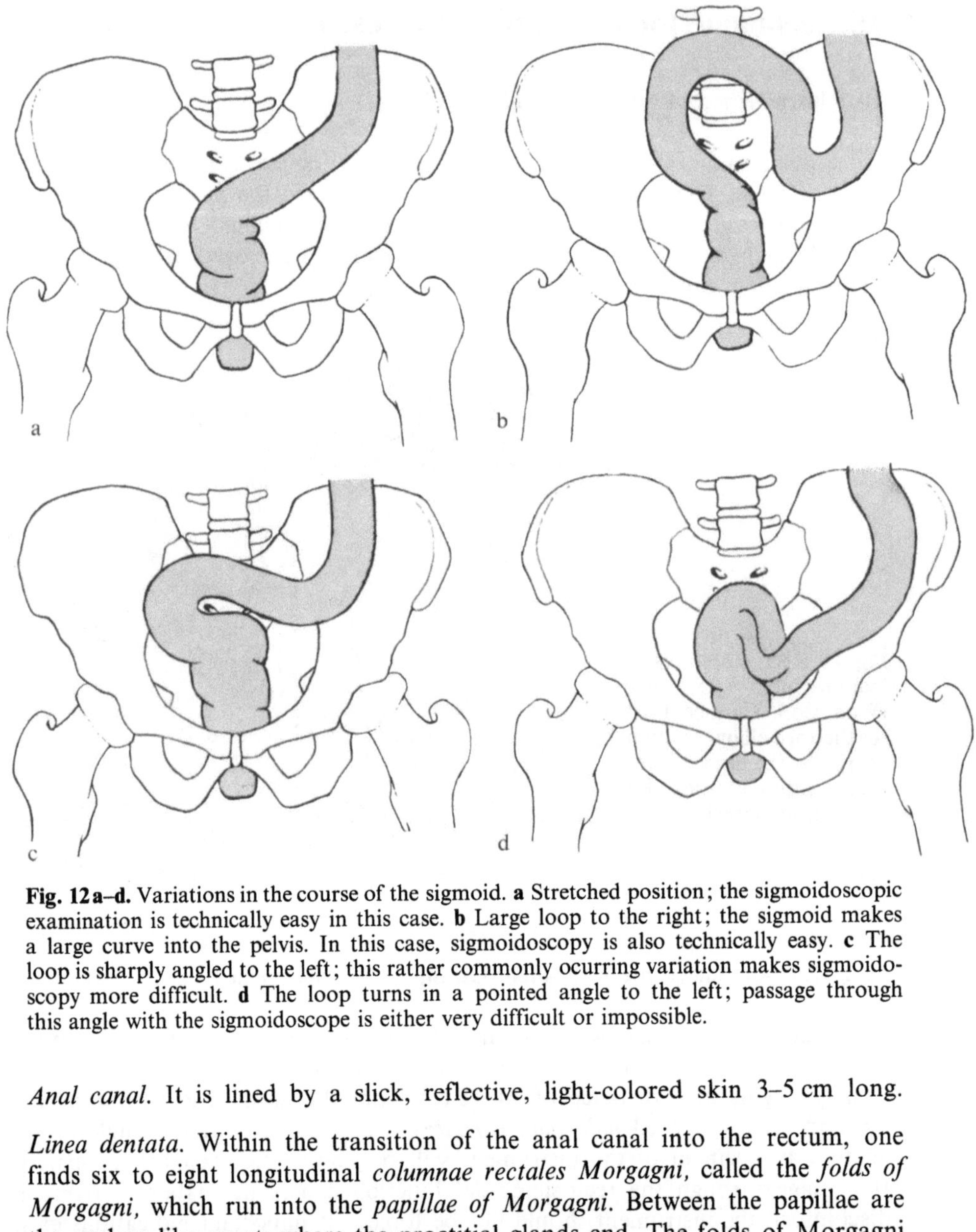

Fig. 12a–d. Variations in the course of the sigmoid. **a** Stretched position; the sigmoidoscopic examination is technically easy in this case. **b** Large loop to the right; the sigmoid makes a large curve into the pelvis. In this case, sigmoidoscopy is also technically easy. **c** The loop is sharply angled to the left; this rather commonly ocurring variation makes sigmoidoscopy more difficult. **d** The loop turns in a pointed angle to the left; passage through this angle with the sigmoidoscope is either very difficult or impossible.

Anal canal. It is lined by a slick, reflective, light-colored skin 3–5 cm long.

Linea dentata. Within the transition of the anal canal into the rectum, one finds six to eight longitudinal *columnae rectales Morgagni,* called the *folds of Morgagni,* which run into the *papillae of Morgagni.* Between the papillae are the syphon-like *crypts* where the proctitial glands end. The folds of Morgagni contain the corpus-cavernosum-like spaces that empty into the hemorrhoidal veins. In cases of *hyperplasia* and *ectasia,* they develop into *hemorrhoids.*

Fig. 13a–d. Schematic representation of the position of the rectoscope in relation to the endoscopic appearance of the bowel. **a** Introduction of the rectoscope in the direction of the umbilicus: view of two semicircular folds, valves of Houston or Kohlrausch; anterior portion of the rectal ampulla. **b** Lowering of the handle; view of the rectal ampulla, posterior portion. **c** Lifting of the handle; rectosigmoid junction at 15 cm. **d** Further penetration with the rectoscope; convoluted sigmoid folds.

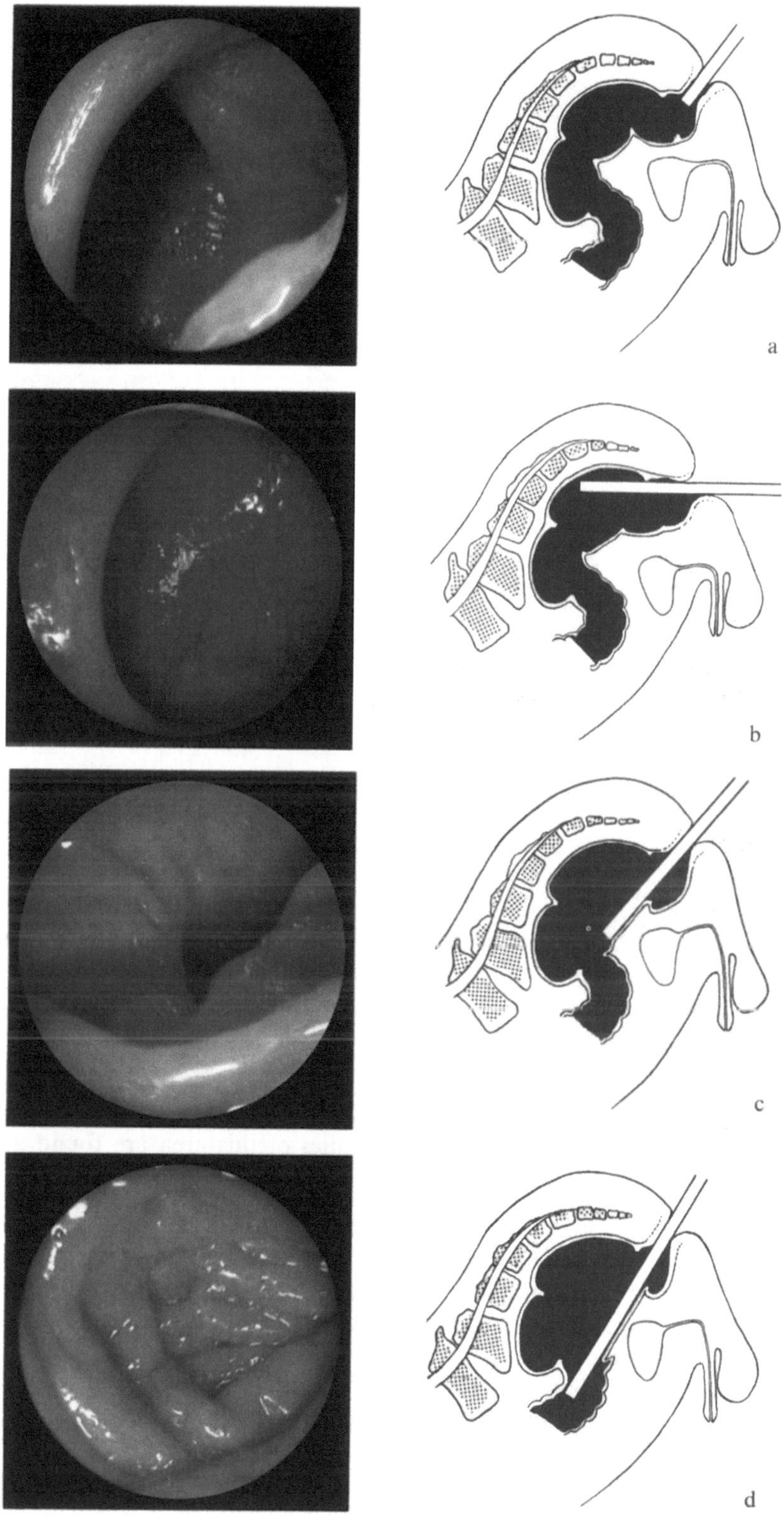
a
b
c
d

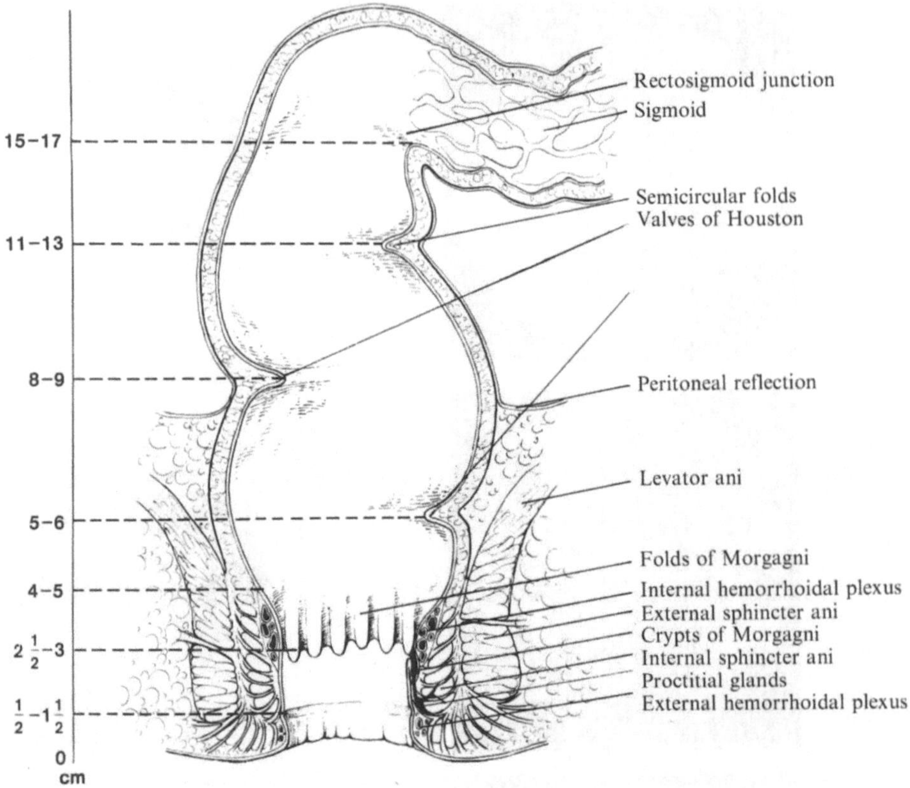

Fig. 14. Topography of the anorectal area.

Ampulla recti. The mucus membrane is slick, light, and interwoven with fine vascular channels (Plate I/1). The filling of these vessels can be influenced by psychological factors, irritation, enemas, laxatives, and spasm. An increased vascularity should not be equated with the presence of inflammation (Plate I/2). Three folds, plicae transversales, traverse the rectum at approximately 7, 9, and 11 cm in a semicircle (*valves of Houston or Kohlrausch*).

Rectosigmoid junction. The characteristics of this area are found at the 15-cm level (14–16 cm). The angle may occur with many individual variations.

Sigmoid. The appearance of the rectum and sigmoid varies considerably depending upon the status of the tone. In most instances, the rectal ampulla is slick while the sigmoid contains convoluted folds. With decreased tone, the sigmoid may even appear tube-like with several semicircularly running folds. The straightening of these folds can be accomplished through the insufflation of air from the attached balloon after closing the rectoscope window. By this maneuver, which raises intraluminal pressure, the elasticity and any deformation of the wall of the bowel can be determined (*"pneumokinetic endoscopy"*).

The actual diagnostic examination occurs during withdrawal of the instrument in a circular fashion permitting all areas to be evaluated. *"Blind spots"* are situated dorsally just behind the *linea dentata.* This region is, however, also accessible to the finger. On the other hand, it is possible that abnormal findings, especially small tumors, may be hidden behind the semicircular plicae transversales.

10.4 Factitial Lesions due to Patient Preparation and Examination

Artificial lesions may be caused by nonprofessionally administered enemas. These lesions often appear as semicircular *'bleeding lines".* The mucosal interruption caused by the introduction of the instrument can lead to bleeding, particularly when passage through the rectosigmoidal junction must be accomplished by a small amount of force. This finding is without significance and should not be confused with the increased friability of the mucosa present in patients with ulcerative colitis that bleeds with the slightest touch of a tampon.

During the introduction of a *thermometer* or *clysis* for cleansing the bowel, small ulcers or erosions may develop that are usually located ventrally in the midline (Plate I/3–5).

10.5 Incidental Findings

10.5.1 Melanosis Coli

With laxative abuse using herbal laxatives, the mucosa takes on a *brownish-black* discoloration that is *spotty or leopard skin-like* (Plate II/1 and 2). In early cases, the lymph follicles only appear whitish through the mucous membrane. Although this picture may be endoscopically quite impressive, it does not have clinical significance and is reversible. In association with *laxative abuse of long standing,* damage occurs in the ganglion cells, the muscularis mucosa, and the muscularis propria, which may lead to atony of the colon. *The presence of melanosis coli should induce the physician to make the patient aware of the consequences of laxative abuse.*

10.5.2 Colica Mucosa ("Mucus Colitis")

The statement by the patient that *mucus* or *connected mucus strands* have been passed through rectum is in itself not infrequently an indication for performing rectoscopy. In these patients, the examiner only sees a somewhat edematous mucosa. These changes can be regarded as reflecting an irritable bowel that is not identical with an inflamed bowel. The term "colitis" in this context is wrong.

10.6 Biopsy

10.6.1 Forceps Biopsy

Direct biopsies from *circumscribed lesions* may be obtained with forceps. Mucosal biopsies with forceps are preferably taken from the semicircular folds. A biopsy from the flat mucosa is difficult to obtain. As the forceps do not cut sharply, the biopsy specimen must be twisted from the mucosa. In cases of *diffuse* mucosal disease, such as inflammation or amyloidosis, use of the *suction biopsy* is preferable.

10.6.2 Suction Biopsy (Plate I/6)

With the *rigid biopsy probe* after Heinkel, it is sometimes difficult to line up the opening of the suction biopsy capsule with the bowel mucosa. This can be more easily done with the *flexible biopsy probe* after Ewe (Fig. 7b).

The biopsy probe is attached to a suction pump with a suction capacity of approximately 500 mm Hg and is inserted through the rectoscope. When the whistling noise accompanying suction stops, the mucosa has been drawn into the biopsy capsule opening and the cutting device is used. Suction is also possible with a 50 or 100 ml syringe.

10.7 Complications

10.7.1 Perforation

Perforations with the suction biopsy capsule have not yet been described. *With forceps biopsy, the mucosal biopsy should, if possible, be taken from the posterior wall distal to the rectosigmoid junction.* With biopsies taken from beyond this region, perforation may lead to the development of peritonitis, particularly when bleeding from the biopsy site must be controlled by electrocoagulation. Nonsurgical treatment using antibiotics usually proves to be adequate for the management of most of these cases.

The reported incidence of complications with rectoscopy is around 1:10,000–20,000, the majority of which are perforations.

10.7.2 Bleeding

Bleeding after biopsy is usually minimal and responds to conservative treatment.

Management. In most instances bleeding can be stopped by the use of compression with *cotton swabs soaked in adrenaline.* If the bleeding continues, *electrocoagulation* of the site must be performed. Some biopsy forceps have an insulated shaft and can be used for electrocoagulation. Only in very exceptional cases is surgical intervention necessary. In any case, control of bleeding will be easier when the biopsy has been taken from an area not higher than 8–10 cm above the anus.

10.8 Removal of Polypoid Lesions (Fig. 15)

Small polyps up to 0.5 cm in diameter may be removed with the biopsy forceps. Larger polyps should be removed with a polyp snare. Pedunculated polyps

correct

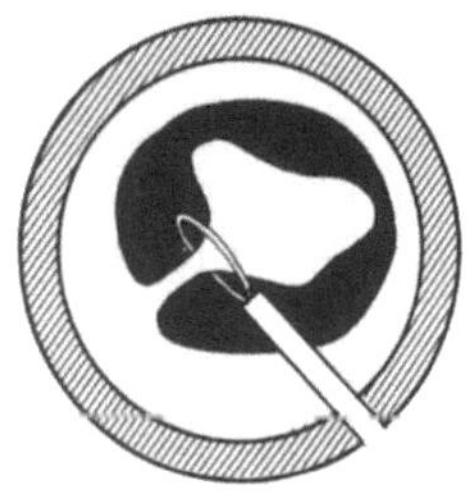

a

Fig. 15a–e. Schematic presentation of the correct (**a**) and incorrect way (**b–e**) of performing snare cautery polypectomy. **a** The snare has been placed optimally around the stalk of the polyp. **b** Incorrect placement of the loop in the middle of the polyp head – danger of severe bleeding due to the opening up of one or more vascular channels. **c** The loop has been placed too close to the base of the stalk. Should bleeding occur after resection of the polyp, electrocoagulation of the site can hardly be done. **d** A portion of the wall of the bowel has also been enclosed within the loop; perforation during resection of the polyp is possible. **e** When contact between the head of the polyp and the contralateral wall of the bowel occurs during electrocautery resection, the danger of perforation exists.

incorrect

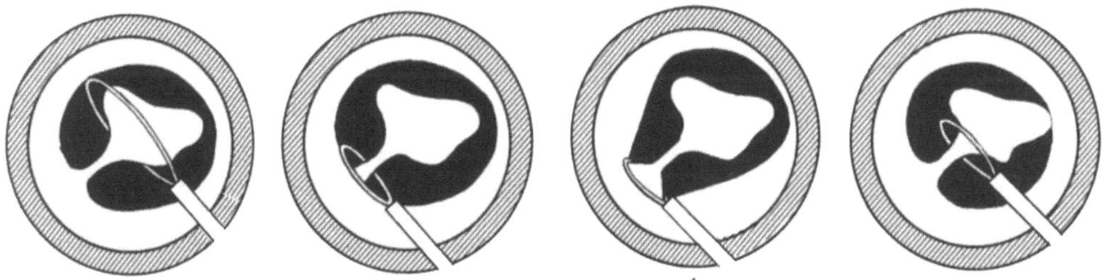

b c d e

can usually be removed on an outpatient basis. *In cases of broad base polyps that are larger than 2 cm in diameter, the polypectomy should be done in a hospital since the danger of postexcisional bleeding increases with the size of the polyp.*

Special preparation of the patient is usually not necessary when a polyp is to be removed from the rectosigmoid region. The polyp is positioned and the polypectomy loop placed around the polyp. It is essential when doing this that no mucosa from the bowel wall be enclosed within the loop. With large polyps that almost entirely fill the lumen of the rectoscope, this can be difficult. The stalk of the polyp should be severed close to the head of the polyp (Fig. 15a) so that in the case of bleeding further resection of the remaining portion of the stalk will permit coagulation (Plate XV/4 and 6).

The loop should then be pulled half open into the rectoscope to free any trapped mucosa from the bowel wall. The loop should be closed and the electrocautery current applied. If it is later noticed that a portion of the polyp remains, this residuum can be removed by a repetition of the technique. The defect in the bowel wall that occurs with polypectomy usually disappears after 2 weeks. The degree of healing should, however, be monitored rectoscopically during this time.

References

Melanosis coli

Buie, L.A.: Practical proctology, 2nd ed. Springfield (Ill.): C.C. Thomas 1960
Henning, N.: Über die Melanosis coli. Z. Gastroenterol. 7, 71 (1970)

Wittoesch, J.H., Jackman, R.J., McDonald, J.R.: Melanosis coli: General review and study of 887 cases. Dis. Colon Rectum *1*, 172 (1958)

Biopsie, Komplikationen

Andresen, A.F.R.: Perforations from proctoscopy. Gastroenterology *9*, 32 (1947)
Barone, J.E., Sohn, N., Nealon, T.F. Jr.: Perforations and foreign bodies of the rectum: Report of 28 cases. Ann. Surg. *184*, 601 (1976)
Haas, P.A.: Darmperforation bei der Proktoskopie. Zentralbl. Chir. *84*, 1207 (1959)
Heinkel, K.: Die Endoskopie und Probeexzision des Enddarmes. Bibl. Gastroenterol *5*, 309 (1962)
Heinkel, K., Elster, K., Henning, N., Landgraf, J.: Die Saugprobeexzision aus dem Rektum. Methodik und morphologische Ergebnisse. Klin. Wochenschr. *38*, 578 (1960)
Haubrich, W.S.: Proctosigmoidoscopy. In: Gastroenterology, 3rd ed. Bockus, H.L. (ed.), Vol. II. Philadelphia: Saunders 1976
Morson, B.C.: Rectal biopsy in inflammatory bowel disease. N. Engl. J. Med. *287*, 1337 (1973)
Neiger, A.: Atlas der praktischen Proktologie. Bern, Stuttgart, Vienna: Huber 1973

Polypectomy

Buie, L.A.: Practical proctology, 2nd ed. Springfield (Ill.): C.C. Thomas 1960
Dietrich, K.F.: Proktologie für die Praxis. München: Lehmann 1969
Jackman, R.J., Beahrs, O.H.: Tumors of the large bowel. Series MPCS *8*. Philadelphia, London, Toronto: Saunders 1969
Neiger, A.: Atlas der praktischen Proktologie. Bern, Stuttgart, Vienna: Huber 1973
Nesselrod, J.P.: Clinical proctology. Philadelphia, London: Saunders 1957

11 Colonoscopy

11.1 Endoscopic Instruments

Flexible instruments that are available for use in examining the large bowel include the *short* fiberscopes (650–1050 mm in length) for *sigmoidoscopy* and the *long* fiberscopes (1250–1865 mm in length) for *colonoscopy*. For the usual circumstances that one encounters in practice the sigmoidoscope will suffice. In this regard, the short sigmoidoscopes with a length of 650–750 mm (F 91 S, American Cystoscope Makers Inc. (ACMI); TCF-IS, Olympus Co., rectosigmoidoscope after Otto, Wolf Co.) are particularly appropriate because of their easy maneuverability. High colonosocopy that requires more personnel and is technically more difficult should be performed in a hospital.

At the present, instruments are available from five firms. Details about these fiberscopes are presented in Table 1. For an optimal examination, it is preferable that the tip of the instrument be maneuverable in two directions since this option offers the only possibility for introducing the fiberscope without other help (guides) through the sigmoid angle with optimal examination of all areas.

The instruments manufactured by the Olympus Co. (Fig. 16) are of excellent quality; with these fiberscopes *air insufflation, irrigation,* and *suction* can be accomplished by finger pressure on two trumpet valves. With the ACMI instruments (Fig. 17), irrigation must be handled by an aide. The Machida, Wolf (Fig. 18), and Storz instruments lack automatic controls, but additional equip-

Table 1. Technical data concerning available sigmoidocolonoscopes.

Type	Olympus[a]			ACMI[a]			Machida[a,b]		Wolf[a,b]			Storz[b] Fiberscope 13210
	TCF 1S	CF/MB$_3$	CF/LB$_3$	F-91-S	F-9-S	F-9-L	FCS-M	FCS	Recto-Sig-moidoscope after Otto 7893	Sigmoido-skop 7895	Colono-scope 7895	
Length (mm)	725	1115	1865	650	1050	1650	740	1830	750	950	1700	1250
Distal diameter (mm)	16	13.5	13.5	15	15	15	14.5	14.5	14.5 conic	15.5–13.5 conic	15.5–13.5 conic	12
Observation range (°)	85	85	85	75	75	75	60	60	70	70	70	60
Deflection range (°)	170 140	180↕ 160↔	180↕ 160↔	150	180	180	120	120	180↕ 160↔	180↕ 160↔	180↕ 160↔	180↕ 90↓ 90↔
Up-down (1st knob)	+	+	+	+	+	+	+	+	+	+	+	+
Right-left (2nd knob)	+	+	+	+	+	+	+	+	+	+	+	+
Fixed focus (mm)	8–100	10–100	10–100	7–100	6–100	6–100	7–45	7–45	5–∞	5–∞	5–∞	3–∞
Air insufflation (automatic)	+	+	+	+	+	+	–	–	–	–	–	–
Suction (automatic)	+	+	+	+	+	+	–	–	–	–	–	–
Suction and irrigation (automatic)	+	+	+	+	+	+	–	–	–	–	–	–

[a] These firms make a double-channel instrument especially constructed for colonoscopic polypectomy:
Olympus TCF/2L (long instrument);
ACMI F-9-R (short instrument) with increased distal diameter to 18 mm;
Machida FCS-M-W (short instrument), FCS-W (long instrument). Wolf catalogue No. 7892 (short instrument).
[b] These firms make additional air insufflation, irrigation, and suction pumps:
Machida AWS (air water suction supply); Storz catalogue No. 13240; Wolf catalogue No. 20 10.000+20 30.31; ACMI 710 air/water source for TFX-Colonoscope (the new series of the TX instruments possess double disks for turning the tip of the instrument as with the Olympus instruments).

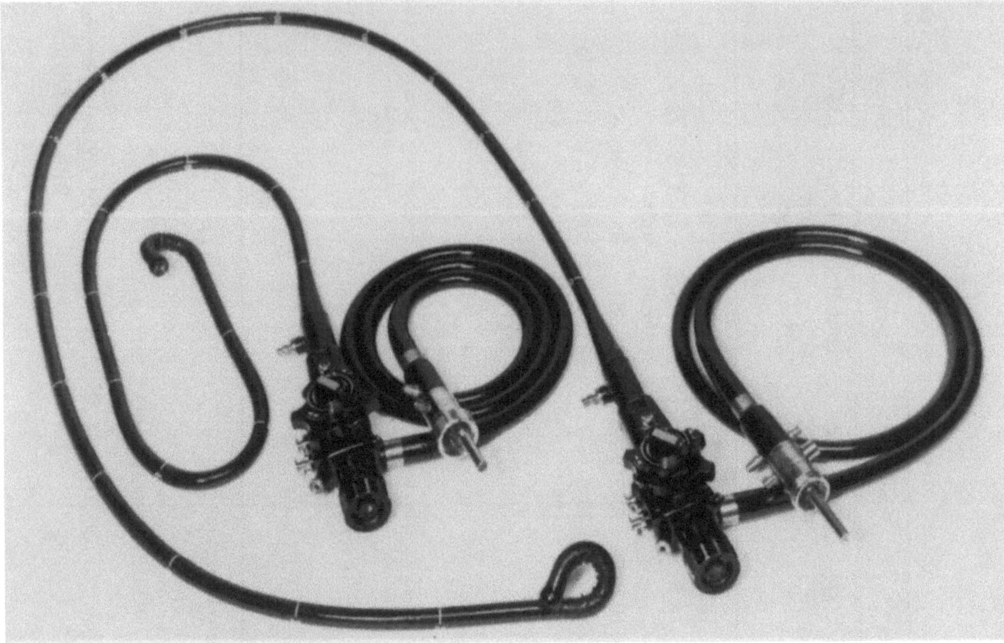

Fig. 16. Colonoscope CF/MB_3 and CF/LB_3 from Olympus Co.

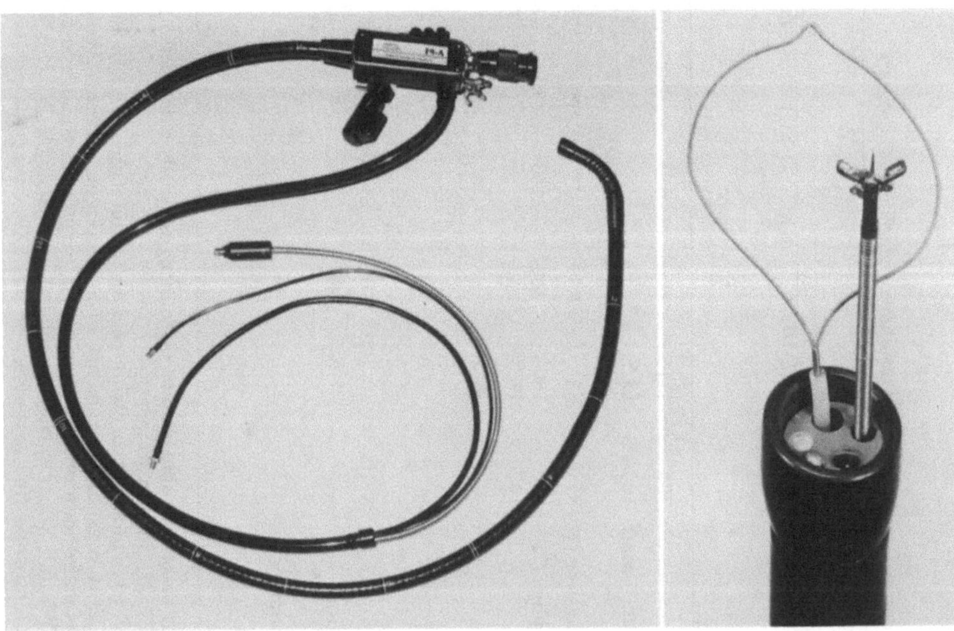

a b

Fig. 17a and b. a Colonoscope F9–A from ACMI. **b** Distal end of the double-channel colonosocope F9-A with penetrating high-frequency diathermy loop (oval) and standard biopsy forceps.

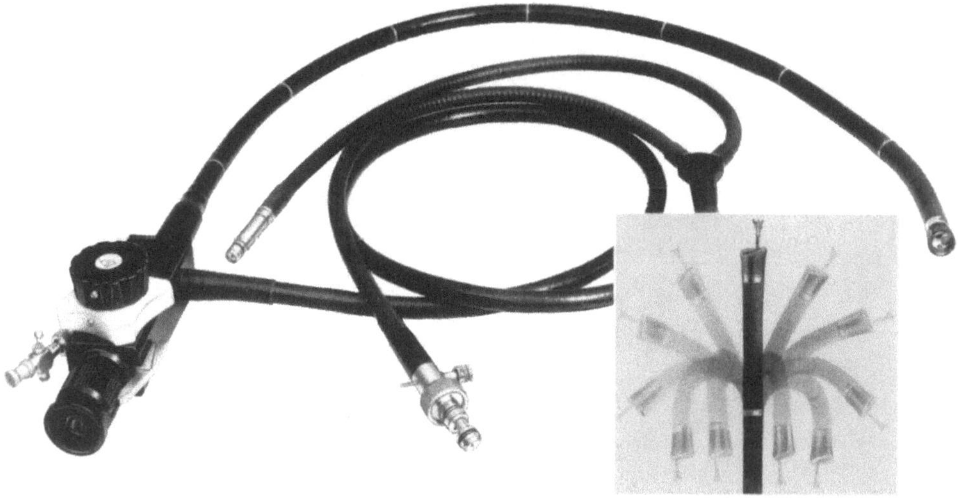

Fig. 18. Rectosigmoidoscope after Otto (7893 from Wolf Co., Knittlingen). Equal movability of the tip to that found in Olympus, ACMI, Machida, and Storz instruments.

ments for air insufflation, suction, and irrigation are offered. The optical quality of the aforementioned instruments is good to excellent.

It is certainly of some advantage in the double-channel Olympus instrument type TCF/2L that the biopsy forceps can be angulated. The second channel in the newer instruments can also prove useful in the performance of endoscopic polypectomy.

11.2 Additional Instruments

"Teaching attachment". Available for the Olympus, ACMI, and Wolf instruments. Is used during sigmoidoscopy by the assistant who is helping to introduce the instrument (see Sect. 11.3 and Fig. 19).

Stiffening rods. Used to stiffen the colonoscope after straightening of the sigmoid loop so that more force can be transferred to the tip of the instrument and advancement can be facilitated (obtainable from ACMI) (Fig. 20).

Plastic sheaths. 40 cm long, which can be passed over the colonoscope and used to maintain straightening of the sigmoid loop (Olympus) (Fig. 20).

Excision biopsy forceps. Used for target biopsy (Olympus, ACMI, Machida, Wolf, Storz) (Fig. 23).

Nylon brush for exfoliative cytology.

Instruments for polypectomy. High-frequency diathermic loops for colonoscopic polypectomy (ACMI, Olympus, Storz, Wolf) (Fig. 21, see also Fig. 17b).

Spiral and asymmetric loops seem to be more advantageous than simple loops when polypectomy is performed. These loops make snaring of the polyp

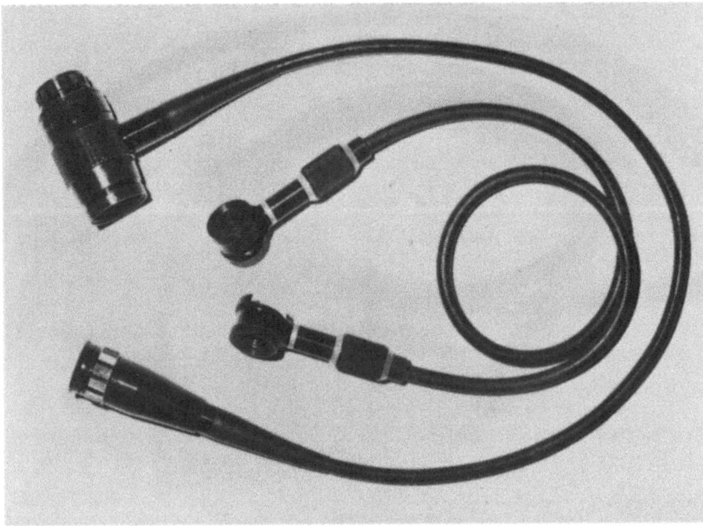

Fig. 19. Teaching attachment (demonstration attachment) from the firms Olympus (*outer*) and ACMI (*inner*).

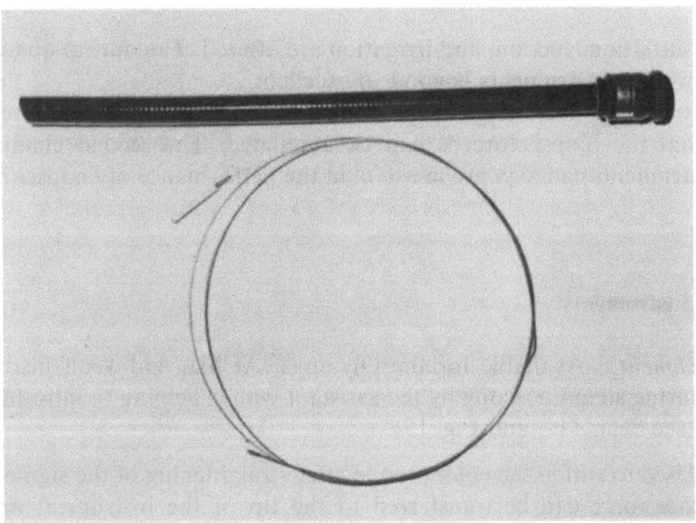

Fig. 20. Stiffening wire for stiffening the colonoscope after straightening of the sigmoid loop (ACMI); similar device also from Wolf, Knittlingen (*below*); stiffening sheath ST-C_3 Olympus Co. (*above*).

easier, and during resection they permit a slower transection of the polyp stalk with a lower risk of postexcisional bleeding.

Modified polyp forceps after Seifert. Used in retrieving the polyp after its excision (Fig. 22).

High-frequency diathermy instruments (Erbe, Tübingen, FRG; Martin, Tuttlingen, FRG) offer a mixture of spark gap and conductive current.

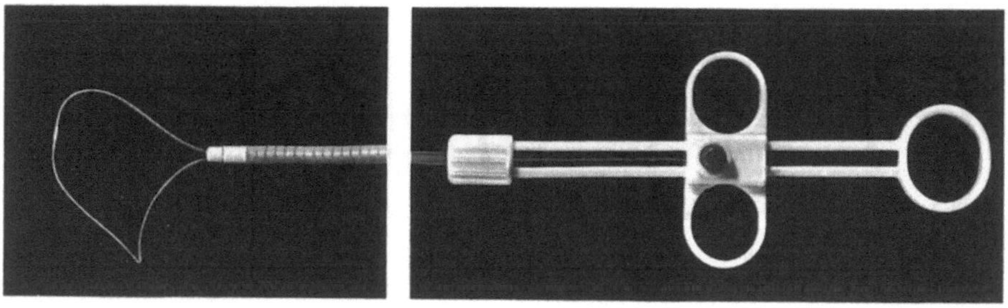

Fig. 21. High-frequency diathermy loop (excentric) (Olympus Co.).

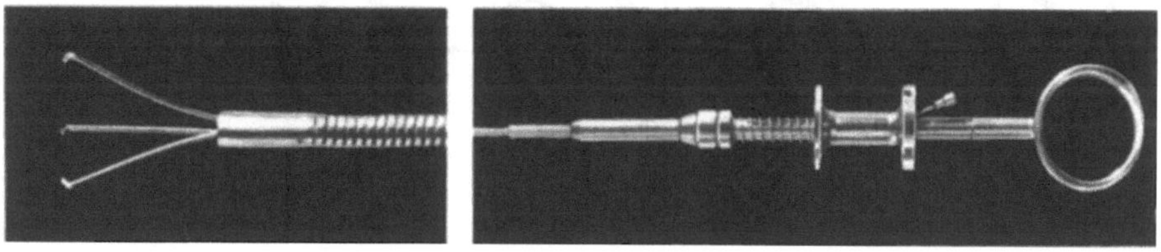

Fig. 22. Polyp retriever forceps (Olympus Co.).

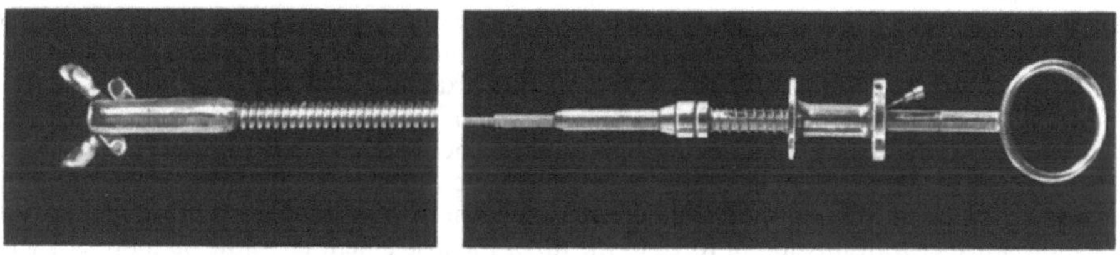

Fig. 23. Standard biopsy forceps with oval spoon (Olympus Co.). The same instrument is also available from ACMI, Machida, Wolf, and Storz.

11.3 Examination Technique

The examination is conducted with the patient recumbent. For sigmoidoscopy some examiners also recommend the knee-elbow or knee-chest position. It is preferable to have two people conduct the examination with the assistant slowly introducing the instrument while observing the field through the *teaching attachment* (see Sect. 11.2).

During high colonoscopy it is usually necessary, especially in the *sigmoid area,* to *straighten* the instrument. This manipulation should be done under X-ray control. For sigmoidoscopy only, X-ray control is not required although the exact location of a lesion may pose a problem when X-ray control is not used.

The *main difficulty* in performing colonoscopy is the passage of the scope through the sigmoid. Because of the poor visibility resulting from the loop formation, passage of the instrument is often done blindly. It is important that the mucosa retains its reddish color and its vascular pattern as the instru-

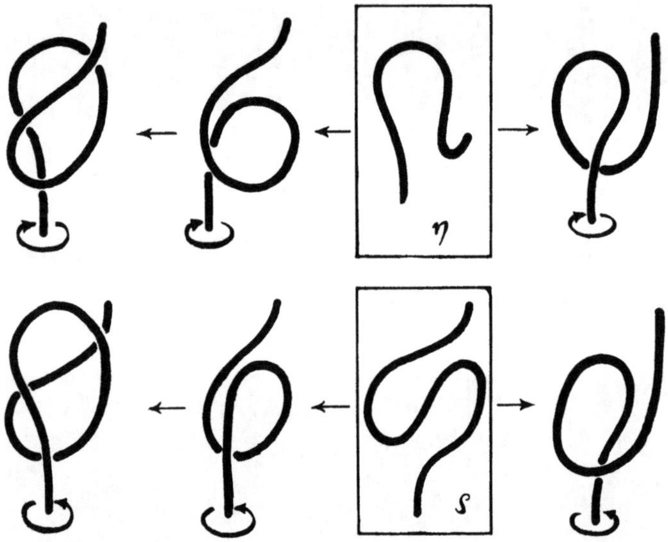

Fig. 24. Schematic presentation of both basic types of sigmoid configuration (η and ς types enclosed in boxes) with their derivations. To achieve straightening of the instrument, the tip of the fiberscope must be at least in the descending colon and better still in the splenic flexure so that the instrument hangs from the distal transverse colon like a walking stick. The examiner should now rotate the instrument on its axis. The loop of the sigmoid is then simultaneously undone by pulling on the instrument and straightening it. After the performance of this maneuver, the examiner will note that all the patient's complaints about discomfort usually cease since the tension on the mesosigmoid has been removed. If an η-type sigmoid configuration is encountered, the instrument can only be advanced to the descending colon or to the splenic flexure, if the fiberscope is then withdrawn 20–30 cm and rotated counterclockwise. The η loop may be converted into an α loop. Further transmission of force to the tip of the instrument can now be more efficiently achieved.

ment *"slides by."* If the mucosa becomes *light red* to *pale* in color or the patient complains about *discomfort*, the instrument must be withdrawn so far that the discomfort subsides and the lumen is visualized. *The discomfort is caused by tension on the mesosigmoid.*

A knowledge of both basic types of sigmoid configuration (very often η and considerably less often ς) facilitates the straightening of the instrument and spares the patient much discomfort (Fig. 24).

Display of the bowel is accomplished through air insufflation and rotation of the patient on the examining table. To avoid abdominal spasm, the amount of air insufflated should be held to a minimum; it is also very difficult to undo a loop formation when the colon is tightly filled with air.

Partial stiffening for straightening of the instrument should be achieved in the sigmoid area through the use of a *stiffening wire* or through insertion of a 40-cm long *plastic sheath* over the bent colonoscope. The experienced examiner should be able to reach the cecum in 30 min. The ileocecal valve is best visualized by angulating the tip of the instrument medially or by inversion in the cecum.

Careful inspection of the bowel should be systematically done after reaching the appropriate colon region and while the instrument is being withdrawn. The biopsy forceps can only be introduced and opened when the instrument is as straight as possible.

The endoscopic picture of the lumen of the colon contains a number of characteristic anatomic features (Fig. 25a–25h). The rectal ampulla is fixed by the perirectal connective tissue and after passage of the instrument through the anal canal, the *cylindric* appearance of this area with the curtain-like folds of Morgagni is observed (Fig. 25a). After passage through the rectum, the tip of the instrument is displaced from its *central-axial* position in the bowel lumen (Fig. 25b) – a semiblind spot. Pushing the instrument towards the descending colon one can recognize the "half moon" appearance of the bowel lumen at the tip of the instrument.

After the instrument has been introduced past the junction of the sigmoid colon with the descending colon, it once again assumes a position in the center of the bowel lumen and the appearance is that of a cylindric bowel lumen. The descending colon is stretched and fixed retroperitoneally so that only minimal insufflation of air is needed for adequate visualization of the lumen. The anatomic angulation of the colon in the splenic and hepatic flexure region also results in a displacement of the instrument from the center of the bowel lumen, which is particularly true for the splenic flexure where there is a *"dome-like roof"* that traps the instrument (Fig. 25e) before it finally passes into the lumen of the transverse colon (Fig. 25f).

The anatomic fixation of the *ascending colon* creates an identical *triangular appearance* of the bowel lumen like that seen in the *descending colon.* In a stretched and widened *ascending colon,* one may see the *cul-de-sac* of the cecum wherein the *cecal pole* is characterized by *converging* folds (Fig. 25g).

11.4 Polypectomy

There is hardly any room for question today about the malignant potential of colon polyps. Therefore, all colon polyps should be removed. The tissue obtained through forceps biopsy of a colon polyp is often *not* representative of the histologic appearance of the entire polypoid lesion. For such a classification, histologic examination of the entire polyp after its complete removal is

Fig. 25a–h. Endoscopic orientation points within the colon; for clarification, the endoscopic findings are compared schematically with the position of the tip of the instrument in the bowel lumen. **a** Rectum: curtain-like folds in the rectal lumen. **b** "Blind area" in the rectosigmoid junction. The appearance of a lumen is lost because the tip of the instrument has been displaced by the acute angulation of the bowel and now lies too close to the bowel wall. Further introduction of the instrument ("slide-by maneuver") is associated with passage of mucosa by the visual field. **c** Half-moon formation. The appearance of the lumen at the junction of the sigmoid colon with the descending colon. **d** Cylindric, triangularly appearing bowel lumen in the descending colon, created by the retroperitoneal fixation of the colon. **e** Dome and second "blind area" in the region of the splenic flexure before the instrument passes into the transverse colon. **f** Cylindric, triangular appearance of the transverse colon. **g** View of the cecal cul-de-sac and cecal pole characterized by converging folds. **h** Ileocecal valve; lip-like form.

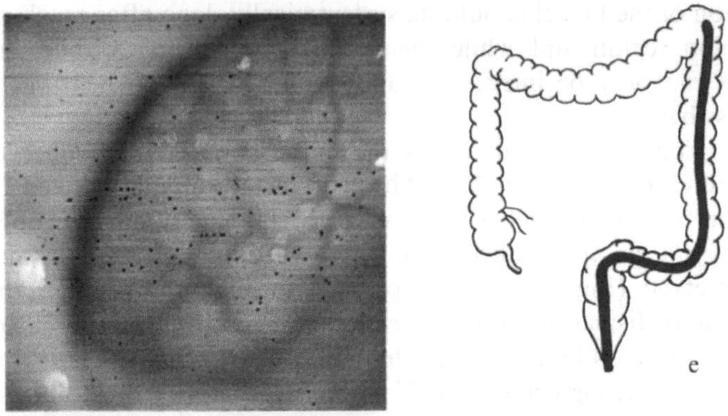

e

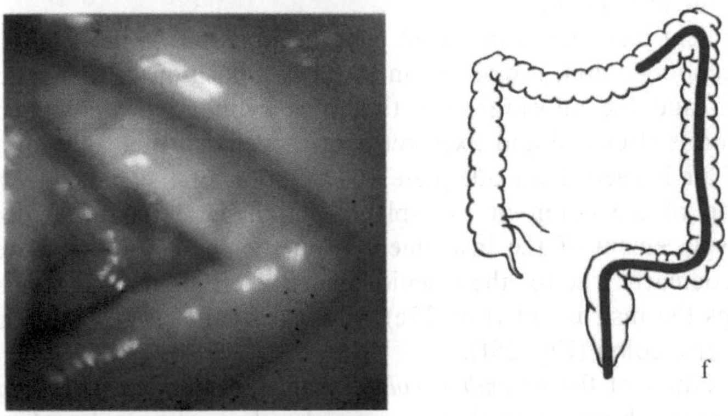

f

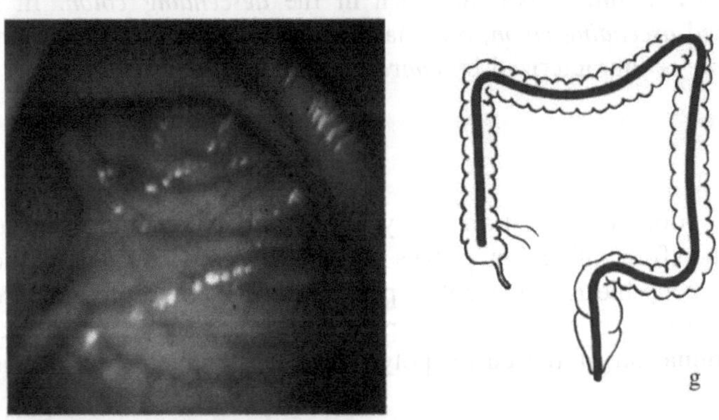

g

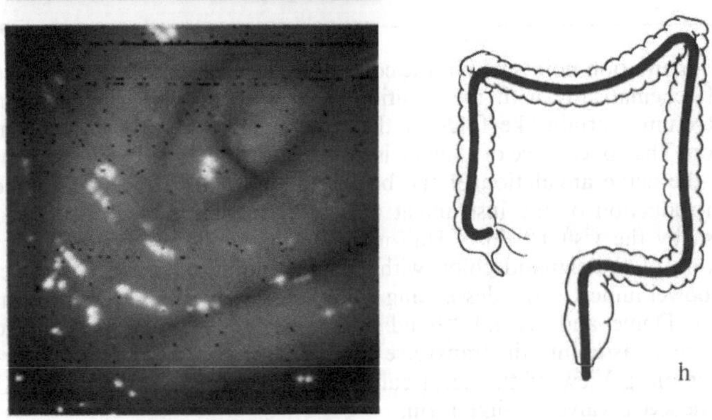

h

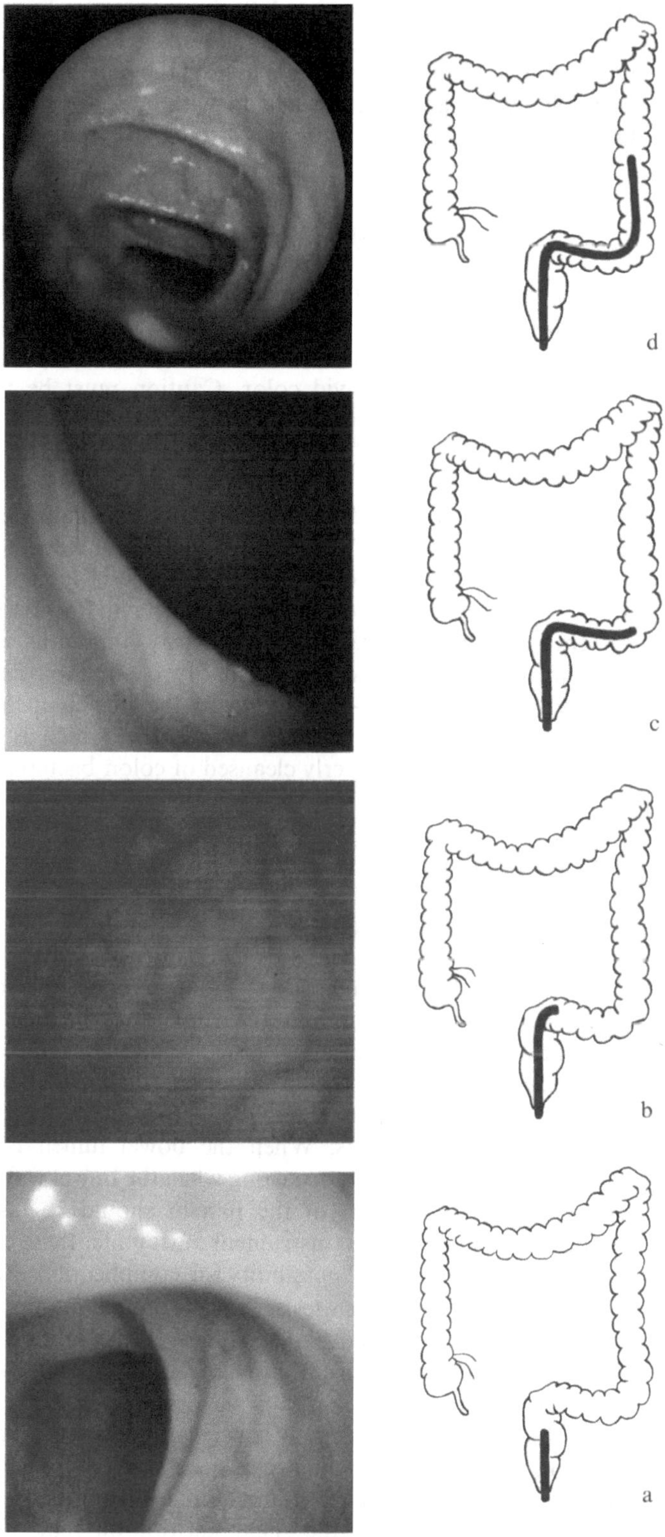
d
c
b
a

mandatory. The polyp removed during colonoscopy should therefore be retrieved. For this purpose, one can either use biopsy forceps or a special polyp retriever. Frequently, it is possible to hold the polyp on the tip of the colonoscope by applying constant suction and to withdraw the polyp with the instrument. Otherwise, the polyp can be retrieved by giving the patient an enema.

11.4.1 Technique of Polypectomy (Fig. 15)

The polyp should be *centrally* placed and the wire polypectomy snare threaded through the instrument channel. The snare loop is extended as far as possible and is placed over the polyp to its base. The loop is then withdrawn until the polyp changes to a livid color. Caution must be taken at this time that *sufficient space* has been left between the loop and the wall of the bowel (*2–5 mm*), otherwise cautery resection of the polyp can lead to perforation. The loop should be visible as far as possible to assure that contact with the wall of the bowel has been avoided. By application of cautery current during simultaneous closure of the loop, the polyp stalk is divided. The current should be applied only over a period of about 2 seconds interrupted by intervals of a few seconds. This will reduce heat damage to the tissue and the danger of perforation. The high-frequency diathermy apparatus is usually set at a dial position of 3–4. To avoid the possibility of an explosion due to the presence of a *mixture of methane-oxygen gas* in the bowel, the resection can be done under *carbon dioxide* or *nitrogen insufflation,* which is, however, unnecessary if the bowel has been properly cleansed of colon bacteria that produce methane.

11.5 Complications

11.5.1 Sigmoidocolonoscopy

Complications during diagnostic sigmoidocolonoscopy seldom occur. The incidence of complications is usually given as 0.2%. The most common complication is perforation. Perforation may occur during the examination of a patient with acute ulcerative colitis or Crohn's disease. The most common site of perforation is in the area of the recto-sigmoid junction or in the flexures because of the blind spots in these areas. When the bowel lumen is not visible, a *whitish discoloration* of the mucosa occurring when the bowel wall slides by accompanied by *discomfort* on the part of the patient should be taken as a warning that perforation is possible. The instrument must under these circumstances be *rapidly* withdrawn. An additional possibility for complication exists when air is *forcibly* insufflated. This usually causes severe abdominal cramping, and prompt utilization of suction will remove the danger of perforation. Special caution must be exercised during the insufflation of air in patients with diverticulosis since the diverticula may be a cause for perforation. A penetration of a diverticulum by the biopsy forceps may also conceivably lead to perforation. Biopsies from a stenotic area of the colon, when necessary, should therefore only be taken from the margin of the diverticulum and not from its base. Fraught with special danger for the patient is the silent perforation that often goes unnoticed by the inexperienced examiner and is detected only hours later after the development of peritonitis and pain.

Deaths due to postoperative complications following laparotomy performed because of perforation are extremely rare (0.03%) and are usually due to myocardial infarction or pulmonary embolus.

11.5.2 Polypectomy

Complications such as perforation, massive hemorrhage from the polyp stalk, and breakage of the polyp snare are infrequent and can be avoided by close attention to the following points:

a) Avoid coagulation disorders either defined by history or laboratory data
b) Slowly electrocoagulate the polyp stalk and avoid too rapid a closure of the snare loop
c) Check all polyp snares before using them
d) Maintain a proper separation (safety distance) between the polyp snare and the bowel wall
e) Do not remove any *sessile* polyps having a diameter greater than 1 cm

The incidence of complications with colonoscopic polypectomy is reported as 1.5% whereby only 0.5% of all such polypectomies require subsequent surgical intervention. Most episodes of bleeding following polypectomy respond to conservative treatment. Blood transfusions are usually not necessary. Mortality rates associated with the transabdominal removal of polyps using a colotomy are in contrast 1.5%–2%.

References

Azukani, P., Paoluzi, P., Capurso, L.: Endoscopy of the colon. Proceedings of the 1st European Congress on Digestive Endoscopy. Prague, 1968. Basel, New York: Karger 1969

Bond, J.H. Jr., Levitt, M.D.: Factors affecting the concentration of combustible gases in the colon during colonoscopy. Gastroenterology *68*, 1445 (1975)

Demling, L., Classen, M., Frühmorgen, P.: Atlas der Enteroskopie. Berlin, Heidelberg, New York: Springer 1974

Demling, L., Frühmorgen, P., Koch, H., Rösch, W.: Operative Endoskopie. Stuttgart, New York: Schattauer 1976

Demling, L., Ottenjann, R.: Endoskopische Polypektomie im Gastrointestinaltrakt. Stuttgart: Thieme 1973

Deyhle, P.: Flexible stealwire for the maintenance of the straightening of the sigmoid and transverse colon during coloskopy. Endoscopy *4*, 36 (1972)

Deyhle, P.: A plastic tube for the maintenance of the sigmoid colon during coloscopy. Endoscopy *4*, 224 (1972)

Deyhle, P., Jenny, S., Säuberli, H.: Koloskopische Polypektomie – Résumé nach 300 Eingriffen. Z. Gastroenterol. *7*, 698 (1976)

Deyhle, P.: Fiberoptic colonoscopy. In: Gastroenterology, 3rd ed. Bockus, H.L. (ed.), Vol. II. Philadelphia: Saunders 1976

Frühmorgen, P., Joachim, G.: Gas chromatographic analysis of intestinal gas to clarify the question of inert gas insufflation in electrosurgical endoscopy. Endoscopy *8*, 133 (1976)

Frühmorgen, P., Zeus, J., Classen, M.: Klinische Wertigkeit der Koloskopie. In: Fortschritte

der gastroenterologischen Endoskopie. Vol. IV, Lindner, H. (ed.). Baden-Baden, Brüssel: Witzstrock 1973
Geenen, J.E., Schmitt, M.G., Wu, W.C., Hogan, W.J.: Major complications of coloscopy: Bleeding and perforation. Am. J. Dig. Dis. *20*, 231 (1975)
Jacobson, W.Z., Levy, A.: Colonoscopic perforation: Its emergency treatment. Endoscopy *8*, 15 (1976)
Nagasako, K., Endo, M., Takemoto, F., Kondo, T., Kimura, K.: The insertion of fibercolonoscope into the cecum and direct observation of the ileocecal valve. Endoscopy *2*, 123 (1970)
Nagasako, K., Takemoto, F.: Fibercolonoscopy without the help of fluoroscopy. Endoscopy *4*, 208 (1972)
Nagasako, K., Yazawa, C., Takemoto, F.: Observation of the terminal ileum. Endoscopy *2*, 45 (1971)
Ottenjann, R.: Colonic polyps and coloscopic polypectomy, Endoscopy *4*, 212 (1972)
Otto, P., Huchzermeyer, H.: Results in coloscopic polypectomy. In: Surgical endoscopy. Seifert, E., Witzstrock, G. (eds.). Baden-Baden, Brüssel 1975
Otto, P., Huchzermeyer, H., Müller, H.: Komplikationen bei der Coloskopie – Ergebnisse einer Umfrage an gastroenterologischen Zentren in der Bundesrepublik Deutschland. In: Fortschritte in der Endoskopie. Kongreßbericht des 9. Kongresses der Deutschen Gesellschaft für Endoskopie. München, 1976. Erlangen: peri med 1976
Otto, P., Huchzermeyer, H., Müller, H.: Erfahrungen bei 528 coloskopischen Polypektomien. 10. Kongress der Deutschen Gesellschaft für Endoskopie. Essen, 1977
Otto, P., Paul, F., Töllner, D.: Gibt es endoskopische Orientierungspunkte im Kolon? In: Fortschritte der Endoskopie. Vol. V, Ottenjann, R. (ed.). Stuttgart, New York: Schattauer 1974
Ragins, H., Shinya, H., Wolff, W.J.: The explosive potential of colonic gas during colonoscopic elektrosurgical polypectomy. Surg. Gynecol. Obstet. *138*, 554 (1974)
Smith, L.E., Nivatvongs, S.: Complications in colonoscopy. Dis. Colon Rectum *18*, 214 (1975)
Sugarbaker, P.H., Vineyard, G.C., Peterson, L.M.: Anatomic localisation and step by step advancement of the fiberoptic colonoscope. Surg. Gynecol. Obstet. *143*, 457 (1976)
Williams, C.B., Muto, I., Rutter, K.R.P.: Removal of polyps with the fiberoptic colonoscope: The new approach to colonic polypectomy. Br. Med. J. *1973 I*, 451
Wolff, W.I., Shinya, H.: Colonofiberscopic management of colonic polyps. Dis. Colon Rectum *16*, 87 (1973)

12 Diseases of the External Anal Area

Diseases of the external anal area may be diagnosed during inspection using good lighting. Because of the variable responses to treatment, the individual diseases should be diagnostically distinguished from one another.

12.1 Eczema (Plate II/3–5)

Acute and chronic anal eczema usually accompanied by very aggravating pruritus ani are common symptoms or consequences of internal hemorrhoids. In this case the disturbed action of the anal sphincter plays an important role. As a result of the constant wetness from the prolapsed tissue, anitis, proctitis, chronic anal fissure or fistula, a continuous irritation develops. Sometimes a fungus infection (especially soor mycoses) may play an etiologic role. Additional considerations include chronic diarrhea, long-term therapy with antibiotics, contact dermatitis resulting from clothing, detergents, and even toilet paper as well as hemorrhoidal salves or suppositories. Swellings in the rim of the anus (hemorrhoidal tags, condylomata, fibromata) may also lead to an eczematous pruritus. Particularly inclined toward the development of eczema are obese patients and those with a funnel-type anus since the massive buttocks and perspiration are predisposing factors. Depending upon the stage and degree of involvement, various manifestations of anal eczema are encountered. With diffuse reddening of the periphery of an erythematous lesion accompanied by fissures, an associated mycotic infection must be considered. Excessive wetness indicates an acute anal eczema. Thickened lichenification of the skin with dryness and hyperceratosis are usual findings with chronic anal eczema.

12.2 Hemorrhoidal Tags (Plate II/6)

An appreciation of *perianal skin tags* is necessary if one is not to confuse these with *external hemorrhoids.* They may be quite variable in size, and in contrast to external hemorrhoids they do *not* fill with pressure. As a result of recurrent inflammation they may be completely fibrosed. They are significant only insofar as they prevent optimal cleaning of the anal ring and thereby may contribute to the development of anal pruritis and eczema. Removal of these tags for cosmetic or hygienic reasons by electrocauterization can be easily done under local anesthesia. Predisposing factors for the development of hemorrhoidal tags may be perianal thrombosis, a stretching of the skin during childbirth, or anal fissures.

12.3 Perianal Thrombosis ("Hematoma") (Plate III/1)

We are referring here to an acutely developing thrombosis in the subcutaneous veins of the anal margin. This relatively frequent and very painful experience for the patient can usually be diagnosed from the medical history. After straining upon defecation, diarrhea, lifting of weights, or without apparent reason, a very painful, pea- to bean-sized, bluish-red knot develops in the anal margin. These sometimes ulcerate spontaneously and precipitate heavy bleeding. Within the differential diagnosis of perianal thrombosis, one must also consider incarcerated prolapsed hemorrhoids, if after incision no thrombus can be extruded.

Without treatment, the swelling may remain for several weeks. The intensity and duration of discomfort will depend upon the size of the thrombosis and the degree of accompanying phlebitis. Pronounced thrombophlebitis can involve the entire anal region. Very edematous lumps often contain multiple thrombi and then require multiple incisions for their treatment. Anal skin tags remain as residua of large sized thromboses.

Treatment (Plate III/2–4). During the first few days, incision can be accomplished without the use of anesthesia. After incision the thrombus is usually extruded. In certain cases, pressure on the vessel will result in still another thrombus. Frequently the injection of local anesthesia is more painful for the patient than a skilled incision alone. The use of a heparin-containing salve after incision, sitz baths, phenylbutazone, or antibiotics locally in the face of marked inflammation may prove helpful. If indicated because of recurrence, excision and removal may be needed.

12.4 External Hemorrhoids (Plate III/5 and 6)

External hemorrhoids are rare but are often diagnosed because patients and many doctors refer to all visible and palpable findings in the anal region as "external hemorrhoids."

External hemorrhoids are covered with skin and appear as soft lumps within the external anal margin that can be emptied out and filled with pressure in contrast to perianal skin tags (Sect. 12.2). They must not be confused with perianal thrombosis and prolapsing internal hemorrhoids, which are always covered by the bowel mucosa.

If external hemorrhoids are found, extensive internal hemorrhoids are usually also present. When the internal hemorrhoids are removed, the external hemorrhoids also disappear.

12.5 Anal Fissure

Next to perianal thrombosis, an anal fissure is the most common cause for a painful process in the external anal area. An anal fissure is a linear ulcer that underlies the fissure adjacent to the internal anal sphincter, which in turn reacts with an increased tone. Causes for an anal fissure include an infected subcutaneous thrombosis and tears in the anal region from hard stools or foreign bodies. It is often not possible, however, to define the precipitating factor.

12.5.1 Acute Fissure (Plate IV/1)

Complaint. Pain, usually sudden in onset following a hard stool or diarrhea and with burning or sticking components. The important historic features here are the association of the pain with defecation and the duration of the pain for several hours thereafter with painful spasm of the anal sphincter. As a consequence of the above, constipation usually follows.

Diagnosis. The fissure will be found in 90% of the cases in the posterior commissure commonly accompanied by a *"sentinel fold"* – an edematous fold where the fissure ends. After spreading the buttocks, the examiner will note a small, linear-oval ulcer with a yellowish-red slimy base ranging in size from a grain of rice to a plum pit. As an acute fissure is accompanied by painful spasms of the sphincter, the rectal examination should be performed under local anesthesia (1–2 ml of a local anesthetic injected with a fine needle into the fissure). General anesthesia is not recommended. After local anesthesia, the sphincter spasm disappears and the examination can be performed without pain or difficulty.

12.5.2 Chronic Fissure (Plate IV/2)

If the acute anal fissure is not treated, it can within the course of weeks or months become chronic. The pain is then not as severe, and the rectal examination is almost always possible without anesthesia. The patient complains about wetness and slime in the anal area, considerable itching with perianal eczema, and blood streaking of the stool. Chronic anal fissures can be distinguished from the acute fissure through their firm undermined borders and in most cases also by their clean base within which the white diagonal fibers of the anal sphincter are visible.

Treatment with the acute fissure. Following the injection of a local anesthetic into the base of the fissure using a fine hypodermic needle, the pain stops immediately and defecation is thereafter practically painless. If the injection is made too deeply, an abscess can result that must then be treated surgically. The formerly practiced stretching of the sphincter under general anesthesia should only be done by experts because of the danger of tearing the anal sphincter with this technique. With the use of the other method given above, stretching is also not necessary.

In the case of a *chronic fissure,* treatment using injections is usually not successful. A longitudinal incision with removal of the undermined margins may performed. The lateral sphinctero-myotomy is usually to be preferred. The use of cortisone-containing salves has proved unsuccessful.

12.6 Condylomata (Plate IV/3,4)

12.6.1 Pointed Condylomata (Condylomata Acuminata)

According to current theories, pointed condylomata are caused by a virus infection. The process can originate from wetness and dampness around the anus. A causal relationship to a veneral disease has not been shown but a side-effect of gonorrhoe is certainly possible.

Condylomata acuminata appear as wart-like, displaceable, finger-like, single, or grass-like, small tumors that are sand-colored and rough. Occasionally they also involve the anal canal. Sometimes they may grow to the size of a bean. Pruritus ani and foul-smelling secretion may be accompanying symptoms.

Treatment. Removal with electric loop or by soaking with 20% solution of *podophyllin* in alcohol after protection of the uninvolved areas by covering them with zinc ointment.

12.6.2 Broad Condylomata (Condylomata Lata) (Plate IV/5 and 6)

Broad condylomata are *pathognomonic for lues.* In contrast to the pointed condylomata, the broad ones are moist, broad-based papules with well-defined infiltration.

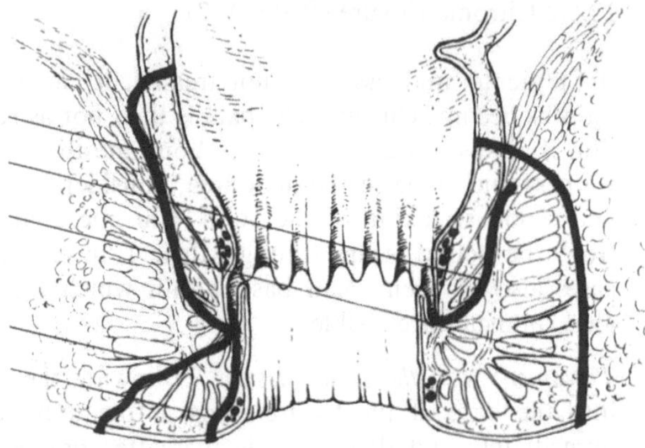

Fig. 26. Schematic presentation of various types of fistulae in relation to the anal sphincters.

12.7 Anal Fistula (Fig. 26 annd Plate V/1–6)

An anal fistula is a chronically infected tract in the anal region that generally does not heal spontaneously. The cause for an anal fistula is almost always an abscess in the anal region arising from a Morgagni crypt or thrombosed and infected hemorrhoid. Anal fistulae are a common complication of Crohn's disease and an infrequent complication of ulcerative colitis. Tuberculosis is recognized as the cause in 1% of the cases. Historically, the initiating cause for a fistula is often an inadequately managed perirectal abscess that spontaneously perforates or after cautious incision has not been opened wide enough to prevent it from reclosing immediately after drainage. The result is an anal fistula.

Depending on the situation and the relation of the fistula to the sphincters, one distinguishes (Fig. 26) between *subcutaneous* or *submucosal, intra-, trans-,* or *extrasphincteric* fistulae or the *ischiorectal* fistula.

For reasons of treatment and prognosis, it is important whether the fistula is *below* or *above* the important closing mechanism of the levator ani muscle in the rectum. The primary fistula opening is located in the anal canal in 90% of cases.

By careful sounding of the outer secondary opening of the fistula (Plate V/1 and 2), the course of the fistula to its primary opening may be determined. It is advantageous to monitor the path of the sound by placing a finger in the rectum for palpation. For orientation, the rule of Goodsall may be used (Fig. 27).

Primary treatment of a perirectal abscess that has been the cause for a fistula should be left to the surgeon who should make as wide an opening as possible and place a long drain in the abscess cavity.

With long-standing chronic fistulae, a thread can be placed to continuously drain the cavity and establish a more favorable basis for surgery. To achieve this, a sound with a perforated tip is used to place the thread through the

Fig. 27. Rule of *Goodsall.* Perianal fistulae whose secondary outer opening lies dorsal to a line running horizontally through the anus have an arch-like tract ending in the anal canal between 11:30 and 12:30 o'clock (knee-elbow position). Fistulae that have an outer opening ventral to this line perianally run straight to the anal canal.

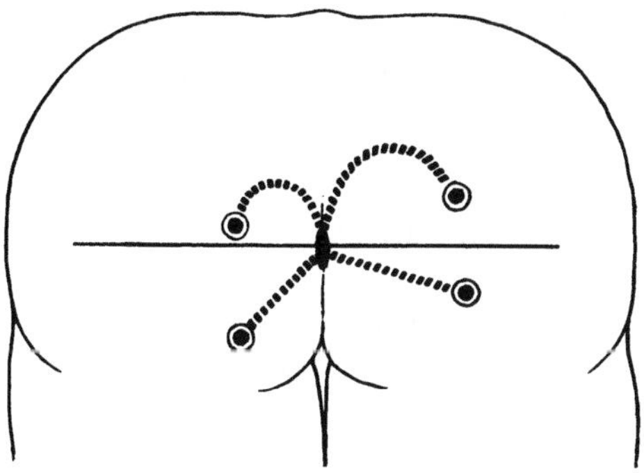

fistula opening. The thread is then brought out through the anus and tied without tension to a ring in front of the outer secondary opening of the fistula (Plate V/4). To assure cleanliness of the anal region, it is advisable that the patient also take sitz baths. With drainage, the massive perianal infiltration quickly disappears and surprisingly the patient does not usually mind the knotted thread. The general health of the patient also improves considerably. This treatment is recommended for the anal fistulae of Crohn's disease since with this condition the underlying disease of the large or small bowel leads to fistula recurrence after surgery.

12.8 Incomplete Fistula (Plate V/5 and 6)

We have purposely separated the incomplete internal intrasphincteric fistulae since they are for the most part undetected and therefore seldom diagnosed. In these cases, the patient often suffers for many years, although when the symptoms are properly recognized such fistulae are easy to diagnose. The important symptom is, in contrast to the pain from a fissure that occurs during defecation, a *delayed discomfort* that occurs 15–20 min after defecation and sometimes lasts for hours (*intermittent pain*). The pain often radiates into the buttocks, hip, or back. Not infrequently, one encounters a macerating eczema with a superimposed mycotic infection.

Diagnosis. On rectal digital examination, small discontinuity of the sphincter can be palpated often, however, with an increased sphincter tone. The lesion is commonly discovered between 11:00 and 1:00 o'clock (knee-elbow position). Often upon spreading the buttocks, a drop or a stream of pus exudes from the anus. This finding along with the classic clinical history is evidence for the existence of an incomplete fistula that can be definitively diagnosed using a speculum and a sound. With this technique using a hook-like sound, the tract running between the internal sphincter area and ending blindly in the external sphincter area under the perianal skin can be followed.

Treatment. The pockets in the skin can be opened with the electrocautery under local anesthesia and the margins removed. Sometimes these can even be torn apart directly with the sound.

Additional treatment. Sitz baths may be helpful. The surgical wound heals very quickly with complete disappearance of symptoms that may have troubled the patient for years.

12.9 Anal Carcinoma (Plate VI/2 and 4)

Of bowel cancers 3%–6% are found in the anus. The problem with this carcinoma is that, although it can be recognized early, it is frequently diagnosed *late* and may have been misdiagnosed as hemorrhoids for weeks, months and even years. *All ulcerating rough anal flaps should, without exception, be biopsied* so that early treatment may be given to the patient. Carcinoma of the anal ring can be excised in otherwise healthy patients together with lymph node dissection of the groins, and postoperative radiation therapy can be given.

12.10 Anal and Rectal Prolapse (Plate VI/1 and 3)

Anal prolapse is characterized by the temporary or permanent protrusion of a part of the rectal mucosa out of the anal canal. Common causes for anal prolapse are advanced hemorrhoids. Grade II and III hemorrhoids prolapse through the sphincter muscle and carry the wall of the bowel with them (*secondary anal prolapse*) (see Sect. 14 and Plate VI/1).

While in the case of an *anal prolapse* only the mucosa and submucosa protrude outward, a *rectal prolapse* contains all the layers of the bowel wall. An anal prolapse resembles a knot with radiating retraction in contrast to the folds that are arranged in a circular manner in the case of a rectal prolapse, which has a telescopic appearance (Plate VI/3).

References

Al-Humadi, A., Alford, J.E.: Sigmoidocervical fistula complicating diverticulitis: Report of a case and review of the literature. Dis. Colon Rectum *17*, 397 (1974)

Ani, A.N., Solanke, T.F.: Anal fistula: A review of 82 cases Dis. Colon Rectum *19*, 51 (1976)

Arnold, K.: Klinik und Therapie des Hämorrhoidalleidens. Langenbecks Arch. Klin. Chir. *332*, 411 (1972)

Bacon, H.E.: Office proctology. Diagnosis and treatment. Postgrad. Med. *53*, 93 (1973)

Böhm, C.: Anorectales Syndrom. Arch. Dermatol. Forsch. *244*, 364 (1972)

Buchan, R., Grace, R.H.: Anorectal suppuration: The results of treatment and the factors influencing the recurrance rate. Br. J. Surg. *60*, 537 (1973)

Dietrich, K.F.: Proktologie für die Praxis. München: Lehmann 1969

Goligher, J.C.: Surgery of the anus, rectum and colon, 2nd ed. London: Baillière, Tindall, Cassell 1967

Homan, W.P., Tang, C., Thorg Jarnarson, B.: Anal lesions complicating Crohn's disease. Arch. Surg. *111*, 1333 (1976)

Keining, E., Braun-Falco, O.: Dermatologie und Venerologie, 2nd ed. Munich: Lehmann 1969

Krause, H., Roschke, W.: Die inkomplette innere Analfistel. Ein nicht seltenes, aber häufig verkanntes Krankheitsbild. Münch. Med. Wochenschr. *107*, 2595 (1965)

Krause, H., Roschke, W.: Die Fadendrainage des perianalen Fistelleidens. Med. Welt *25*, 368 (1974)

Lindell, F.D., Fletcher, W.S., Krippaelme, W.: Anorectal suppurative disease. A retrospective review. J. Surg. *125*, 189 (1973)
Lock, M.R., Thomson, J.P.: Fissure in ano: The initial management and prognosis. Br. J. Surg. *64*, 355 (1977)
Lockhart-Mummery, H.E.: Symposium, Crohn's disease: Anal lesions. Dis. Colon Rectum *18*, 200 (1975)
Lockwood, R.A.: Anorektale Erkrankungen. Stuttgart: Schattauer 1965
Neiger, A.: Atlas der praktischen Proktologie. Bern, Stuttgart, Vienna: Huber 1973
Otto, P.: Die Proktologie ein Stiefkind der Gastroenterologie. Erfahrungen in Diagnostik und Therapie. Z. Gastroenterol. *11*, 107 (1973)
Parks, A.G.: The classification of fistula in ano. In: Progress in Proctology. Hoferichter, J. (ed.). Berlin, Heidelberg, New York: Springer 1969
Parks, A.G., Thomson, J.P.: Intersphincteric abscess. Br. Med. J. *1973/2*, 865, 537
Reeder, D.D., McGehee, R.N.: Office management of pilonidal disease and anorectal lesions. Am. Fam. Physician *8*, 179 (1973)
Roschke, W.: Die proktologische Sprechstunde, 4th ed. München, Berlin, Vienna: Urban & Schwarzenberg 1976
Stelzner, F.: Die anorektalen Fisteln, 2nd ed. Berlin, Göttingen, Heidelberg: Springer 1976
Sumikoshi, Y., Takano, M., Okada, M., Kiratuka, J., Sato, S.H.: New classification of fistulas and its application to the operations. Am. J. Proctol. *25*, 291 (1974)
Tagart, R.E.: Haemorrhoides and palpable anorectal lesions Praetitioner *212*, 221 (1974)
Turrel, R.: Diseases of the colon and anorectum. Vol. 2. Philadelphia, London: Saunders 1959

13 Anitis – Cryptitis – Papillitis

Inflammatory processes within this transitional zone cannot be separated from one another and often occur together. The source of the infection will usually be found in the crypts of Morgagni, originating in the dorsal crypts and spreading to the adjacent papillae. The area of involvement appears erythematous and edematous, and pus occasionally exudes from the crypts. An association exists between cryptitis and the development of anal fissures, and between anal fissures and hemorrhoidal diseases. The anal canal is for the most part also involved in the inflammatory process. One encounters an anitis, which because of an increased secretion produces a perianitis and perpetuates a perianal eczema (Plate VII/1 and 2). Hypertrophy of the papillae then develops (Plate VII/3–6). These changes have also been described with gonorrhea and lues, which can be diagnosed microscopically using a smear or darkfield examination.

Symptoms. Anitis and proctitis are characterized by itching and wetness. In pronounced cases, blood may be noted on the toilet tissue. In cases of cryptitis/papillitis, the patients complain about a mild sensation of pressure in the anal region without a definite relationship to defecation.

Treatment. Using salves and suppositories, the treatment should be initially conservative; the papillae should be soaked with a 10%–20% solution of phenol and glycerin. Inflamed crypts can be incised with the curved knife (cryptotom). Large papillae, especially when they are prolapsing, can be excised with the electric loop (Plate VII/3–6).

14 Hemorrhoids

Hemorrhoids are spongy, blood-containing protrusions just in front of the linea dentata (Figs. 13 and 29). In Germany the observations of Stelzner et al. (1962) have been accepted, which maintain that we are dealing here with hyperplasia and ectasia of a cavernous body, the corpus cavernosus recti, which as part of a continence organ serves an important closing function. Sites of predilection for hemorrhoids are the junctions of the arterial vessels at 2:00, 5:00, and 9:00 o'clock (knee-elbow position). In addition to these main knots, one frequently finds additional knots (Fig. 28). Buie states that over 80% of all people over 30 years of age have hemorrhoids. The presence of hemorrhoids per se does not mean, however, that the patient experiences discomfort. The hemorrhoids are under the control of the visceral nervous system and because of this they are not sensitive to punctures, cuts, or burning. Their removal using rubberband ligation also causes no pain (see Sect. 14.2.3). Other symptoms must be present before we recognize a "hemorrhoidal disease." The typical symptoms of hemorrhoids, perhaps also caused by associated anitis or papillitis, are those of wetness, itching, and burning in the anus in addition to a pressure sensation (see also Sect. 13, cryptitis). Blood, usually bright red in color, may also be noted around the stool or on the toilet paper.

14.1 **Staging** (Plate VIII/1–4 and Fig. 29)

Stage I. The most common finding is that hemorrhoids prolapse or protrude into the proctoscope and tend to bleed (Plate VIII/1 and 4).

Stage II. Hemorrhoids prolapse and protrude after defecation but retract spontaneously. Since fibrosis has begun, the tendency to bleed is less (Plate VIII/2).

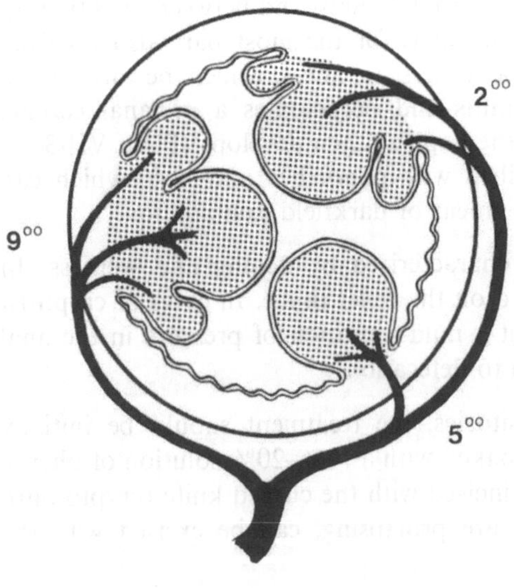

Fig. 28. Schematic representation of the arterial vasculature of the hemorrhoidal knots (knee-elbow position). Arising from the branches of the arteria rectalis superior, which lies at the level of the linea dentata (5 cm distance from the anal ring), these protrude at 2:00, 5:00, and 9:00 o'clock. Through further branching of the vessels at 2:00 and 9:00 o'clock, additional so-called satelitic knots may develop.

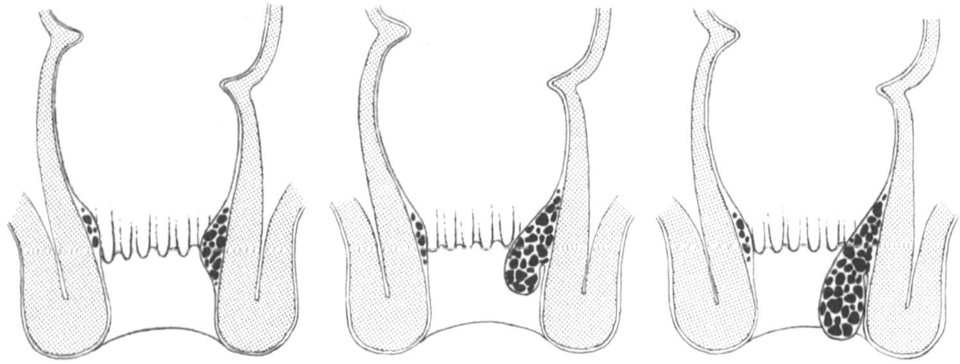

Fig. 29. Schematic presentation of hemorrhoid staging.

Stage III. Hemorrhoids prolapse more pronouncedly but can usually be replaced with the finger. The tendency to bleed is slight (Plate VIII/3).

Fibrosis occurs in the course of time with stage II and especially stage III hemorrhoids and their prolapse then responds hardly, if at all, to replacement. Synonymous with stage II and III hemorrhoids are replaceable anal prolapse (stage II hemorrhoids) and unreplaceable hemorrhoids and partially replaceable or secondary anal prolapse (stage III hemorrhoids).

14.2 Treatment

1. Symptomatically with suppositories

2. Sclerosing treatment (Plate VIII/5 and Fig. 30). The success rate for sclerosing treatment of stage I hemorrhoids is excellent and with stage II good. These cases should not be operated since the success rate with sclerosing is equally as good, if not better, than with surgery. Stage III hemorrhoids, especially those with a fixed anal prolapse, are clearly surgical problems. If the patient refuses surgery, an attempt with sclerosing may be made, since it is often possible to achieve significant subjective improvement, and sometimes even a partial retraction of the prolapse occurs.

Sclerosing treatment *after Blond:* A 20% solution of quinine (Sagitta proct., Sagitta-Werk/Munich, FRG; quinine-HCl, Buchler/Braunschweig, FRG) is injected dropwise through the side window of the proctoscope only into the submucosa at the base of the hemorrhoid knots. Per session up to 1 ml of quinine solution is injected. If the needle is too close to the surface of the bowel, necrosis may occur, and if it is too deep, the bowel musculature will be injected instead of the hemorrhoids. If the position of the needle is not known with certainty, then one should inject only a small amount of the solution. The presence of an increased resistance indicates that the needle is in the musculature. Particular precautions must be taken with injections in the ventral region.

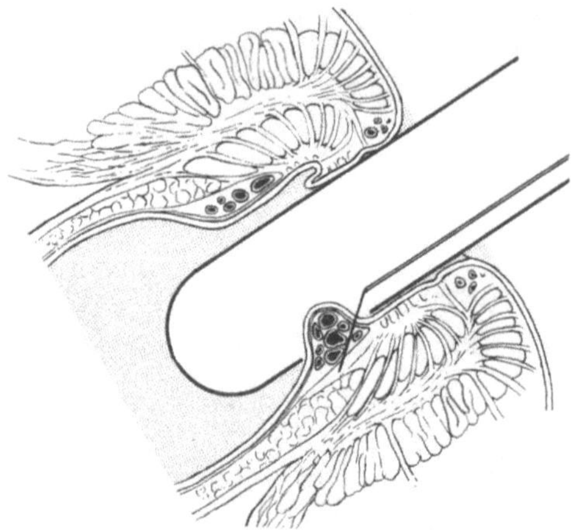

Fig. 30. Schematic presentation of the sclerosing technique of Blond

The frontal commisure should be avoided. Injection into the prostate will cause the patient discomfort and into the urethra will produce dysuria.

Because of the vascularity, the chance of the injection causing an infection is slight and desinfection of the injection site is not necessary.

When turning the proctoscope, one must be careful not to drag along the injected hemorrhoid with the instrument causing the same area to be injected twice. The bleeding from the injection site is not of significance and severe bleeding will not be encountered. As a rule, five to eight injections in weekly intervals will suffice for lasting success.

Sclerosing treatment *after Bensaude:* Using *sodium tetradexylsulfate solution* 0.5–1.0 ml per hemorrhoid knot, two knots at a time may be treated, and three to four injections at weekly intervals are usually sufficient.

Sclerosing treatment *after Blanchard:* In this case a total of up to 10 ml of a 5% phenol solution in oil is injected submucosally under the hemorrhoid knots until the mucosa blanches and the capillaries become prominent. As a rule two to three injections are sufficient to relieve the patient of his discomfort.

Contraindications to the use of sclerosing treatment: With acutely inflamed processes, hemorrhagic diathesis, and during pregnancy (quinine) hemorrhoids should not be injected. In 1% of patients an allergy to quinine exists. An ulcer after superficial injection may also occur (Plate VIII/6).

3. Ligation with rubberbands using special instruments may be performed whereby the elastic band is put around the hemorrhoid. The hemorrhoid is thus devascularized and will fall off within a few days.

4. Thermocoagulation by the infrared coagulator (Neiger).

5. Operation. Usually the three-tip method of Milligan and Morgan or a modification of this technique by Parks is preferred.

References

Bensaude, R., Bensaude, A.: Les hemorroides et leur traitement. In: Maladies de l'intestin, 5th ed. Vol. IV. Paris: Masson 1939
Blond, K., Hoff, H.: Das Hämorrhoidalleiden. Leipzig, Vienna: Deuticke 1936
Böhm, C.: Das Hämorrhoidalleiden. Stuttgart: Schattauer 1967
Dietrich, K.F.: Proktologie für die Praxis. München: Lehmann 1969
Editorial: What are haemorrhoids. Brit. Med. J. *1975/3*, 354
Haas, D.: Rektosigmoidnekrose nach Haemorrhoidalverödung. Helv. Chir. Acta *43*, 591 (1976)
Hansen, H.H.: Neue Aspekte zur Pathogenese und Therapie des Hämorrhoidalleidens. Dtsch. Med. Wschr. *102*, 1244 (1977)
Held, H., Heilmann, S.: Chininspiegel im Serum bei der Hämorrhoidenverödung nach Blond und Hoff. Phlebol. Proktol. *5*, 156 (1976)
Jeffery, P.J., Parks, A.G., Ritchie, J.K.: Treatment of haemorrhoids in patients with inflammatory bowel disease. Lancet *1977/I*, 1084
Müller, J.M., Fiedel, G., Stock, W., Pichlmaier, H.: Die Gummibandligatur, eine Alternative bei der Behandlung des Hämorrhoidalleidens. Dtsch. Med. Wochenschr. *101*, 1798 (1976)
Neiger, A.: Atlas der praktischen Proktologie. Stuttgart, Bern, Vienna: Huber 1973
Neiger, A.: Haemorrhoiden: Erkennung und heutige Behandlungsmöglichkeiten. Schweiz. Med. Wochenschr. *108*, 500 (1978)
Otto, P.: Das Haemorrhoidalleiden. Bemerkungen zur Ätiopathogenese, Diagnose und Therapie. Z. Haut- Geschlechtskr. *50*, 315 (1975)
Otto, P., Wettengel, R.: Blutgasanalysen des Hämorrhoidalblutes. Ein Beitrag zur Diskussion über eine arterielle oder venöse Versorgung des Corpus cavernosum recti. Phlebol. Proktol. *1*, 254 (1972)
Pichlmaier, H.: Komplikationen nach Verödungsbehandlung von Hämorrhoiden. Dtsch. med. Wschr. *103*, 408, (1978)
Roschke, W.: Die proktologische Sprechstunde, 4th ed. Munich, Berlin, Vienna: Urban & Schwarzenberg 1976
Steinberg, D.M., Liegeois, H., Alexander-Williams, J.: Long-term review of the results of rubber band ligation of internal haemorrhoids. Br. J. Surg. *62*, 144 (1975)
Stelzner, F.: Die Hämorrhoiden und andere Krankheiten des Corpus cavernosum recti und des Analkanals. Dtsch. Med. Wochenschr. *88*, 689 (1963)
Stelzner, F., Staubesand, J., Machleidt, H.: Das Corpus cavernosum recti – die Grundlage der inneren Hämorrhoiden. Langenbecks Arch. Klin. Chir. *299*, 302 (1962)
Wienert, V.: Ambulante Hämorrhoidektomie durch elastische Ligaturen: Eine Literaturübersicht. Fortschr. Med. *95*, 1619 (1977)

15 Inflammatory Bowel Diseases

The endoscopic aspects of an *inflammatory* colon disease do not permit the differentiation of a nonspecific proctitis from a bacterial enterocolitis and an *ulcerative proctitis.*

Endoscopic findings in colitis

Vascular pattern	Completely absent in acute cases; slurred and irregular in chronic, less florid cases
Surface	Granular, uneven, with dispersed light reflex and increased redness (especially with florid cases)

Friability	Increased with bleeding at the slightest touch, often punctiform
Edema	Folds are thickened and edematous
Secretions	Pus and/or mucus
Ulceration	Ulcerative colitis: flat erosions; not always present Crohn's disease: circumscribed, occasionally as aphtous ulcer or deep ulcers in otherwise normally appearing or minimally altered mucosa
Localization	Ulcerative proctitis-colitis: in rectum alone or in association with colon above Crohn's disease: rectum often not involved, proximal colon involved

The distinction is also aided by the follow-up and bacteriologic examination. In the case of Crohn's colitis, other characteristics peculiar to this disease, when present, assist in the differentiation.

Symptoms. The most indicative symptom of an inflammatory large bowel disease is the passage of blood, mucus, and possibly pus mixed in the stool or the same without the stool. In the case of an isolated proctitis, the bowel habits are not affected. In cases of ulcerative colitis, we mostly find bloody mucopurulent diarrhea. In cases of Crohn's disease, the passage of blood in uncommon.

15.1 Nonspecific Proctitis

It is apparently possible that inflammatory changes in the crypt-papillae-hemorrhoid area may also affect the rectum. Sometimes, however, no cause for the proctitis can be found and no specific symptoms exist. The separation of *ulcerative proctitis* as a special form of ulcerative colitis is certainly not always possible. Nonspecific proctitis may be considered when the history is that of a rapidly healing process (Plate IX/1–3).

15.2 Infectious (Entero-) Proctocolitis

Agents such as *salmonella, staphylococcus,* certain strains of E. coli, some viruses, and others may also produce colitis as a part of the generalized acute intestinal disturbance associated with the infection (vomiting, diarrhea, fever) that resolves without specific treatment. This colitis cannot be distinguished from ulcerative colitis endoscopically. This also applies to the *amebic colitis* wherein we may, however, find many punctate pinhead-sized ulcers covered with pus and a more or less inflamed surrounding mucosa (Plate X/1–6).

15.3 Radiation Proctitis (Plate IX/4–6)

Radiation treatment of malignant tumors within the male or female urogenital tracts using either X-rays or radium can lead to an actinic damage within the adjacent rectal mucosa. This damage manifests itself as bloody stools and in some cases cramping in the rectal area. These symptoms appear within a few weeks or months but sometimes several years following radiation therapy.

Because of increased friability and bleeding tendency, one appreciates with difficulty that the mucosa of the ventral wall of the bowel at the 8-cm level is thickened with a whitish discoloration (Plate IX/4). To exclude an extension of the malignant process into the rectum, it is advisable to watch out for any signs of infiltration and to obtain mucosal biopsy specimens during rectoscopy. Only in rare cases, however, will malignant infiltration be found.

The most important aspect of treatment here is the reassurance of the patient that the symptoms are not caused by a carcinoma. The symptomatic management then includes the use of steroid-containing retention enemas, azulfidine suppositories, antispasmotics, and analgetics.

15.4 Ischemic Colitis – Pseudomembranous Colitis (Plate XIV/3 and 4)

Ischemic colitis has been considered by Marston during the last few years to represent a separate clinical entity. With transient disturbances in blood flow through the region supplied by the inferior mesenteric artery, often without any demonstrable anatomic obstruction, the mucosa of the bowel undergoes necrosis and the underlying layers of the bowel wall remain intact. This results in the sudden occurrence of bloody diarrhea and often abdominal pain in the left side. The differential diagnosis must therefore include acute diverticulitis. The splenic flexure and descending colon are common areas for involvement by ischemic colitis. The rectum is, as a rule, not involved.

Colonoscopy (Plate XIV/4) reveals a pale, necrotic mucosa that later with denudation resembles ulcerative colitis. In the course of events, the mucosa undergoes extensive regeneration and a late complication may be segmental stenosis of the bowel.

In the acute stage of ischemic colitis, the diagnostic considerations also include pseudomembranous colitis (Plate XIV/3), which may arise with long-term treatment using antibiotics. This condition resolves itself after discontinuation of the antibiotics. In the acute stage, mucus and blood may be observed in the stool.

15.5 Ulcerative Colitis

Rectoscopy is the most important diagnostic procedure for the determination of ulcerative colitis because the changes are so clearly seen with endoscopy.

Ulcerative colitis *begins in the rectum* and has the tendency to spread *upward* in the bowel. In a large percentage of cases (60%), the disease is localized in the rectum and sigmoid colon.

The disease process is restricted mainly *to the mucosa.* If crypt abscesses are present in the mucosal biopsy, this finding will support the diagnosis. Changes within the vascular pattern, increased friability, and erythema of the mucosa are not recognizable on X-ray examinations.

The *radiologic examination* of the colon is more complicated, more troublesome for the patient, more expensive, and less informative. Barium contrast examination is only indicated if the extent of the disease involvement is not known or a carcinoma located above the reach of the rectoscope is to be excluded. As an alternative to the X-ray examination, one may elect to use colonoscopy, which in cases of chronic ulcerative colitis can be performed with little difficulty since the colon is atonic and shrunk. In patients with chronic ulcerative colitis that has been present for over 10 years and involves the greater part or whole colon, the risk of developing a carcinoma of the colon is strikingly increased.

15.5.1 Hemorrhagic ("Ulcerative") Proctitis

Ulcerative proctitis is a common *special form* of *ulcerative colitis* and is the least severe form. Restricted, as a rule, to the rectum, ulcerative proctitis spreads up to the colon in only 10% of the cases, and an increased risk of developing a colon carcinoma does not exist. Besides symptoms of bleeding and mucus in the stool, patients with ulcerative proctitis have no other symptoms. The inflammatory process does *not* extend *beyond* 14 cm, and the line of demarcation is usually sharp. A case of universal ulcerative colitis may go into remission through the stage of an ulcerative proctitis.

15.5.2 Active Ulcerative Colitis (Plate XI/2–5)

The major changes encountered in cases of ulcerative colitis with activity are: *dusty red-colored surface, extensive tendency to bleed upon touching the mucosa, edema of the mucosal folds, increased mucus or pus, and erosions.* Deep ulceration is not found with ulcerative colitis but is typical for Crohn's disease.

15.5.3 Chronic Ulcerative Colitis (Plate XI/6; XII/1–5)

The rectoscopic aspects of a *chronic,* mild form of ulcerative colitis in remission *differs* in several points from the findings in acute cases. The normal vascular pattern is destroyed and absent; the mucosa is no longer *erythematous* but is paler; *friability of the mucosa is only slightly increased;* islands of mucosa remain as *pseudopolyps* or inflammatory hyperplasia; the colon wall is relatively stiffened (this can be demonstrated by "pneumokinetics," by changing the lumen with air insufflation).

15.6 Crohn's Disease (Plate XIII/1–6; XIV/1 and 2)

In contrast to *ulcerative colitis, Crohn's disease* may also involve the small intestine, especially the terminal ileum. When the colon is also involved, the tendency exists, in contrast to ulcerative colitis, for involvement to extend distally. The rectum is frequently spared or contains only minimal evidence of the disease.

The following changes may be regarded as evidence of Crohn's disease of the colon: *anal lesions* (in up to 80% of cases) with large, livid fissures that are often symptom-free; *fistulae in ano; aphtous-like lesions* or *solitary ulcers in otherwise normally appearing mucosa; deep longitudinal ulcers* either in slightly or greatly inflamed mucosa; *minimal* signs in the *rectum; obvious changes in the proximal colon and the ileum.*

The biopsy taken from the lesions contains in around 30% of cases the characteristic epitheloid cell granuloma with Langhans' giant cells. A further histologic feature that distinguishes Crohn's disease from ulcerative colitis is the presence of submucosal inflammatory changes. In a small percentage of patients with Crohn's disease and a normally appearing rectal mucosa, the biopsy will nevertheless still show microscopic changes compatible with Crohn's disease. For this reason, a rectal biopsy should be obtained when suspicion exists.

References

Alexander-Williams, J., Steinberg, D.M., Fielding, J.S., Thompson, H., Cooke, W.T.: Proceedings: Perianal Crohn's disease. Endocrinology *95*, 822 (1974)

Baker, W.N.W., Milton-Thompson, G.J.: The anal lesion as the sole presenting symptom of intestinal Crohn's disease. Gut *12*, 865 (1971)

Crohn, B.B., Ginzburg, L., Oppenheimer, G.D.: Regional ileitis: A pathological and clinical entity. J. Am. Med. Assoc. *99*, 1223 (1932)

Dyer, N.H., Stansfeld, A.G., Dawson, A.M.: The value of rectal biopsy in the diagnosis of Crohn's disease. Scand. J. Gastroenterol *5*, 491 (1970)

Fahrländer, H.: Colitis ulcerosa und Enterocolitis regionalis Crohn. Gemeinsames und Unterschiede. Med. Klin. *70*, 1583 (1975)

Farmer, R.G., Brown, C.H.: Ulcerative proctitis: Course and prognosis. Gastroenterology *51*, 219 (1966)

Homan, W.P., Tang, C., Thorgjarnarson, B.: Anal lesions complicating Crohn's disease. Arch. Surg. *111*, 1333 (1976)

Janowitz, H.D., Sachar, D.B.: New observations in Crohn's disease. Annu. Rev. Med. *27*, 265 (1976)

Jeffery, P.J., Parks, A.G., Ritchie, J.K.: Treatment of hemorrhoids in patients with inflammatory bowel disease. Lancet *1977/I*, 1084

Krauspe, C., Müller-Wieland, K., Stelzner, F. (eds.): Colitis ulcerosa und granulomatosa. München, Berlin, Vienna: Urban & Schwarzenberg 1972

Lennard-Jones, J.E., Cooper, G.W., Newell, A.C., Wilson, C.W.E., Avery-Jones, F.: Observations on idiopathic proctitis. Gut *3*, 201 (1962)

Lennard-Jones, J.E., Lockart-Mummery, H.E., Morson, B.C.: Clinical and pathological differentiation of Crohn's disease and proctocolitis. Gastroenterology, *54*, 1162 (1968)

Lockart-Mummery, H.E., Morson, B.C.: Crohn's disease (regional enteritis) of the large intestine and its distinction from ulcerative colitis. Gut *1*, 87 (1960)

Lockart-Mummery, H.E., Morson, B.C.: Crohn's disease of the large intestine. Gut *5*, 493 (1964)

Lockart-Mummery, H.E.: Symposiumon Crohn's Disease: Anal Lesions Dis. Colon Rectum *18*, 200 (1973)

Otto, P., Huchzermeyer, H., Müller, H.: Makroskopische Befunde und histologisches Korrelat bei entzündlichen und tumorösen Dickdarmerkrankungen. In: Fortschritte der gastroenterologischen Endoskopie. Lindner, H. (ed.). Baden-Baden, Brüssel: Witzstrock 1976

Radiation Colitis

Bosch, A., Frias, Z.: Complications after radiation therapy for cervical carcinoma. Acta Radiol. [Ther] (Stockh.) *16*, 53 (1977)
Buie, L.A.: Practical proctology, 2nd ed. Springfield (Ill.): C.C. Thomas 1960
Kawarda, Y., Brady, L., Matsumoto, F.: Radiation injury to the large and small intestines. Am. J. Proctol. *25*, 49 (1974)
Schmitz, R.L., Chao, J.H., Bartolome, J.S.: Intestinal injuries incidental to irradiation of carcinoma of the cervix of the uterus. Surg. Gynecol. Obstet. *138*, 29 (1974)

Ischemic Colitis

Baas, E.U.: Die ischämische Colitis. Dtsch. Med. Wochenschr. *100*, 1247 (1975)
Ewe, K., Baas, E.U.: Durchblutungsstörungen des Gastointestinaltraktes. Acta Gerontol. *7*, 135 (1977)
Lux, G., Frühmorgen, P., Zeus, J., Phillip, J.: Ischämische Kolitis-Amöbenkolitis-Strahlenkolitis. Differentialdiagnostische Aspekte. Z. Gastroenterol. *7*, 695 (1976)
Marston, A.: Clinical features of ischemic colitis. Proc. R. Soc. Med. *59*, 882 (1966)

Infections Proctocolitis

Berkowitz, D., Bernstein, L.H.: Colonic pseudopolyps in association with amebic colitis. Gastroenterology *68*, 786 (1975)
Dritz, S.K., Ainsworth, T.E., Back, A., Boucher, L.A., Garrard, W.F., Palmer, R.D., River, E.: Patterns of sexually transmitted enteric disease in a city. Lancet *1977/II*, 3–4
Gupta, S., Shorma, C.W.: Massive necrosis and perforation of the colon in amebiasis. Am. Surg. *41*, 429 (1975)

16 Parasites (Plate XIX/6)

As an incidental finding during rectoscopy, one may on occasion encounter parasites. *Most often* these are *oxyuris,* less commonly ascaris or other helminths.

17 Diverticulosis — Diverticulitis (Plate XIV/5 and 6)

A diverticulum is defined as an outpocketing of all layers of the bowel wall. In the case of the large bowel, however, the diverticula are the so-called *pseudodiverticula* since here there is a herniation of the mucosa rather than an outpocketing of the entire bowel wall. As a cause for this herniation, both inherited tissue defects as well as muscular hyperactivity in the bowel wall may play a role. The diet may also be a possible contributory factor since low residue-containing foods increase the segmentation of the sigmoid.

Diverticulosis is present in 6%–25% of people, increasing with age until in the 70-year-old group the incidence is 40%. The *most common site for occurrence is the sigmoid colon* (40%), where a special weakness exists in the bowel wall and there are many vascular penetrations. During rectoscopic examination, one almost *never* substantiates the presence of diverticula. With colonoscopy the pockets are often easily recognized. In the case of diverticula with very narrow openings, however, they may not be appreciated during colonoscopy and the barium enema examination is needed for their identification. Diverticula may create a problem during colonoscopy since the risk of perforation of their thin wall with air insufflation or biopsy always exists (Plate XIV/6).

The consequence of chronic diverticulitis is a hypertrophy of the muscularis with a thickening of the colon wall and a narrowing of the bowel lumen. The differentiation of this segmental narrowing, which occurs in 5%–10% of cases from an associated colon carcinoma, is practically impossible on radiologic grounds alone. In situations of this kind, the use of colonoscopy and biopsy of the area of narrowing is particularly warranted. With progressive narrowing of the bowel lumen, it becomes increasingly more difficult to reach the area of stenosis, and the sampling error during biopsy is increased with poor visualization. One should also keep in mind that a biopsy taken inadvertently from the base of the diverticulum may lead to perforation. Due also to the increased danger of perforation, the acute phase of diverticulitis is generally regarded as a contraindication for colonoscopy.

References

Arfwidson, S.: Pathogenesis of multiple diverticula of the sigmoid colon in diverticular disease. Acta Chir. Scand. [Suppl.] *342* (1965)

Cooper, W.L.: Sigmoidoscopic findings that suggest diverticulitis. Dis. Colon Rectum *1*, 120 (1958)

De La Vega, J.M.: Diverticular disease of the colon. In: Gastroenterology, 3rd ed. Bockus, H.L., Vol. II. Philadelphia: Saunders 1976

Pross, E.: Zur Koinzidenz Sigma – Karzinom – Sigmadivertikulitis. Therapiewoche *22*, 1595 (1972)

Reifferscheid, M.: Kolondivertikulitis. Aktuelle Probleme der Diagnostik und Therapie. Symposion Aachen, 1973. Stuttgart: Thieme 1974

18 Tumors

Common to all tumors of the large bowel is their polypoid appearance. The gross appearance, however, does not correlate well with the histologic findings nor the malignant potential. Because of the morphologic variation also found in these tumors, biopsy specimens may not be representative of the entire lesion.

The increased incidence of colon carcinoma in association with colon polyps and the localization of up to 80% of all polyps and carcinomas of the colon in the rectosigmoid region gives strong support for a connection between these lesions and for a precancerous nature of colon polyps. The size of the polyp and its histologic characteristics play a significant role in the determination of the risk of malignancy. In the case of villous adenomas, the risk of malignancy is increased independent of the size of the lesion. With polypoid lesions greater than 2 cm in diameter, the incidence of malignancy is 50%.

18.1 Benign Tumors

Hyperplastic-metaplastic or inflammatory "pseudopolyps" and juvenile polyps as well as hamartomas do not undergo malignant transformation. All polypoid adenomas should be considered to have a malignant potential, and all cases of polyposis should be regarded as frankly precancerous.

18.1.1 Hyperplastic Polyps (Plate XV/1)

In the case of hyperplastic polyps, we are dealing with a broad-based growth, ranging in size from a grain of rice to a pea, with a slick surface having the same color as the adjacent mucosa. Occasionally these lesions may reach the size of 10 mm in diameter. They are characterized histologically by the overgrowth of colon epithelial cells with ectatic crypts. Grossly similar but in their color somewhat lighter than the surrounding mucosa and appearing as a submucosal tumor are the lymphoid hyperplastic polyps. These are composed of one or more hyperplastic lymphoid follicles.

Both of these types are a reaction to mucosal irritation such as infectious diarrhea. They may develop singly or multiply and may recede spontaneously. They are always benign. Their presence, however, does not exclude the simultaneous existence of adenomatous polyps. Since small adenomatous polyps cannot be distinguished grossly from hyperplastic polyps, they should be removed and examined microscopically.

18.1.2 Tubular Adenoma

Adenomatous polyps are neoplastic lesions with malignant potential. A dedifferentiation of the epithelium is characteristic of a polypoid adenoma, but this finding should not be regarded as having the same degree of significance as carcinoma. Only after infiltration and extension beyond the muscularis mucosa is present should one speak of carcinoma. To make this distinction, it is therefore necessary for the pathologist to examine the entire lesion and not multiple biopsy specimens. With a histologic report that only focal carcinoma without infiltration of the polyp stalk exists, the polypectomy can be regarded as curative and as being prophylactic against the later development of carcinoma.

The WHO terminology distinguishes between dysplasia of 1st, 2nd and 3rd degree the latter corresponding to "carcinoma in situ".

18.1.2.1 Papillary Adenoma

These are most often pedunculated, seldom broad-based, polyps with a slick, flappy surface. They may reach a size that fills the entire colon lumen. Their distinction from villous adenomas may sometimes be difficult. With increasing size, they carry a greater risk for malignancy and for this reason should be removed to permit their exact histologic classification (Plate XV/2–6, XVI/1,2, and 4).

18.1.2.2 Villous Adenoma (Plate XVI/3)

Due to their extreme tendency for malignant degeneration (around 30% become malignant at sizes under 1 cm in diameter), these polyps assume a special position. They are localized almost exclusively to the rectosigmoid region, appearing endoscopically as a broad-based, soft, frawn-like emminence. These polyps are very friable in character. The recurrence rate after their removal is high and in 20% of cases one finds invasive carcinoma. Local excision of these lesions by the surgeon is therefore the treatment of choice. Sigmoidoscopic removal may be tried in poor-risk patients when regular follow-up at 6-month intervals is possible (Plate XVI/3).

18.1.2.3 Mixed Forms

The larger papillary adenomas often also show histologic features of villous adenomas, which is a further argument for their complete prophylactic removal since the villous adenoma (see Sect. 18.1.2.2) has a great tendency to become malignant. Endoscopically, these mixed forms can hardly be separated macroscopically from the papillary adenoma.

18.1.3 Familial Polyposis (Adenomatosis) (Plate XVII/1–4)

Familial polyposis, a dominantly inherited illness, is considered to be a frankly precancerous condition. For every 100 patients with colon polyps there is 1 patient with familial polyposis. The condition usually develops after puberty, and the number of broad-based polyps may vary between comparatively few and a complete involvement of the whole colon by numerous, broad-based, half-spheric lesions in close proximity to one another. On occasion, one also finds larger pedunculated adenomas. Because of the extraordinarily great malignant potential of these lesions – by 40 years of age almost all patients with familial polyposis will develop a colon carcinoma – total colectomy is the treatment of choice. When less than 20 polyps are found in the rectum, an ileosigmoidostomy can be performed, the polyps in the rectum removed endoscopically, and the patient closely followed. When more than 20 polyps are present in the rectum, long-term follow-up has shown that the majority of these patients will develop rectal carcinoma. In these cases, therefore, a primary proctocolectomy is preferable.

The *Gardner syndrome,* a variant of familial polyposis in association with mesenchymal tumors in other organs, also has a great tendency toward the development of malignancy. In the Gardner syndrome in addition to diffuse colon polyposis, there are mesenchymal tumors such as: fibroma, lipoma of the skin, osteoma in the maxilla, skull, and long bones.

18.1.4 Peutz-Jeghers Syndrome (Plate XVII/5 and 6)

The Peutz-Jeghers syndrome is an intestinal polyposis with skin pigment flecks especially around the nose and lips. The polypoid lesions in this syndrome are classified as hamartomas and are histologically characterized by a branch-like splintering of the muscularis mucosa. These polyps therefore appear endoscopically as branch-like polypoid lesions split apart. They are found most often

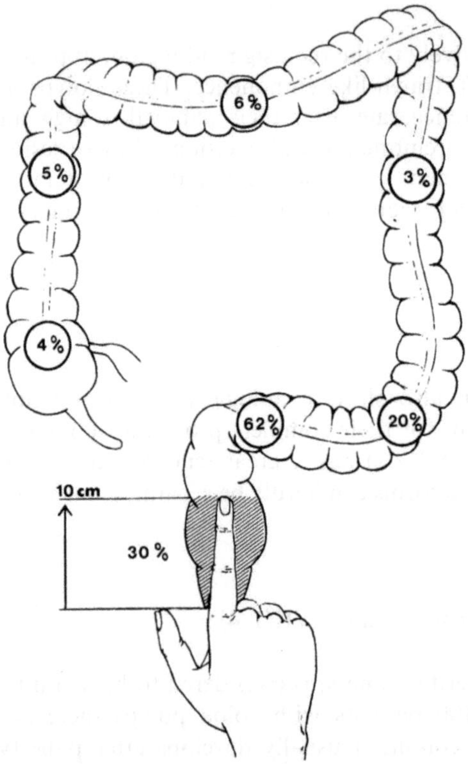

Fig. 31. Localization of large bowel carcinomas. More than 50% are found in the rectosigmoid area. Around one-third of the rectal carcinomas but only one-tenth of all colorectal carcinomas can be detected on digital rectal examination according to Bokelmann et al. (1972).

in the upper gastrointestinal tract. In around half the cases the colon is also involved. The hamartomas are benign. It is noteworthy, however, that individuals with the Peutz-Jeghers syndrome and associated intestinal malignancies develop these bowel cancers 10 years earlier than the normal population. These malignancies do not generally arise from the Peutz-Jeghers polyps themselves.

18.2 Malignant Tumors

The colorectal carcinomas represent the second most commonly occurring carcinomas in the human. More than 60% of these carcinomas arise in the rectum and lower sigmoid region and are therefore accessible to diagnosis with the rectoscopic examination. More than one-third of the rectal carcinomas are present less than 10 cm distant from the anal ring and thus are detectable in the digital rectal examination (Fig. 31).

Endoscopically, one must distinguish between the *cauliflower-like exophytic* lesion that grows stiffly into the bowel lumen and stenoses late (Plate XVIII/1) and the *circumferential* tumor (Plate XVIII/2) that stenoses the bowel early.

One notes endoscopically in the case of the circumferential tumor that the bowel wall is stiff and markedly changed in color, occasionally containing a lumpy necrotic area with increased friability. Often the passage of the endoscope becomes difficult because of a narrowing of the bowel lumen caused by the carcinoma. If the instrument is forced under these circumstances, perforation of the brittle tumor and the infiltrated surrounding tissue may occur.

A distinction between stenosis due to carcinoma and stenosis resulting from inflammation may not always be endoscopically possible. The same applies to small carcinomas on protruding folds, particularly in the areas of the bowel flexures (Plate XVIII/3). Biopsy of the mucosa assumes more than usual importance in these cases when macroscopically the diagnosis cannot be made with certainty. Additionally, neoplastic infiltration from malignancies in adjacent organs (Plate XVIII/4) or infiltration with systemic diseases (Plate XVIII/5 and 6) are not macroscopically definable.

References

Bokelmann, D., Drüner, H.U., Schulz, U.: Klinik und Prognose der Kolon- und Rektumkarzinome. Dtsch. Med. Wochenschr. *97*, 1590 (1972)

Bussey, H.J.R.: The long-term results of surgical treatment of cancer of the rectum. Proc. R. Soc. Med. *56*, 494 (1963)

Decosse, J.J., Adams, M.B., Condon, R.E.: Familial polyposis. Cancer *39*, 267 (1977)

Deyhle, P., Jenny, S., Fumagalli, I.: Endoskopische Polypektomie im proximalen Kolon. Dtsch. Med. Wochenschr. *98*, 219 (1973)

Dischler, W., Oehlert, W.: Dickdarmpolypen – Histologische und endoskopische Klassifizierung und Wertigkeit. Z. Allgemein. Med. *20*, 912 (1974)

Dodds, W.J., Schulte, W.J., Hensley, G.T., Hogan, W.J.: Peutz-Jeghers Syndrome and Gastrointestinal Malignancy. Am. J. Roentgenol. *115*, 374 (1972)

Dozois, R.R., Judd, E.S., Dahlin, D.C., Bartholomew, L.G.: Peutz-Jeghers Syndrome: Is there predisposition to development of intestinal malignancy? Am. Arch. Surg. *98*, 509 (1969)

Eder, M., Wiebecke, B., Klein, H.J.: Pathologisch-anatomische Aspekte der Krebsvorstufen des Gastrointestinaltrakts. Chirurg *41*, 97 (1970)

Elster, K.: Histopathologie der tumorösen Colonerkrankungen. Leber Magen Darm *3*, 111 (1973)

Erbe, R.W.: Inherited gastrointestinal-polyposis syndromes. N. Engl. J. Med. **294**, 1101 (1976)

Feuerle, G.E., Baldauf, G., Hoepker, A.: Acht Jahre Gardner Syndrom in einer Familie. Dtsch. Med. Wochenschr. *102*, 1678 (1977)

Haubrich, W.S., Berk, E.: Malignant tumors of the colon and rectum. In: Gastroenterology, 3rd ed. Bockus, H.C., Vol. II. Philadelphia: Saunders 1976

Inze, F.: The biological significance of rectal polyps. A comprehensive study of 425 cases. Am. J. Proctol. *25*, 49 (1974)

Klostermann, G.F.: Pigmentfleckenpolypose. Stuttgart: Thieme 1960

Langenberg, A.V., Ong, G.B.: Carcinom of large bowel in the young. Br. Med. J. *1972/III*, 374

Loehlein, D., Ziegler, H., Pichlmayr, R.: Polypose des Dickdarms. Ein Vergleich der familiären mit der nichtfamiliären Form. Chirurg *47*, 439 (1976)

Lowe, W.C.: Neoplasma of the gastrointestinal tract. Bern, Stuttgart, Vienna: Hubert 1972

McKittrick, J.E., Lewis, W.M., Doane, W.A., Gerwig, W.H.: The Peutz-Jeghers syndrome: Reports of two cases, one with 30 year follow-up. Arch. Surg. *103*, 57 (1971)

McSherry, G.K., Cornell, G.N., Glenn, F.: Carcinoma of the colon and rectum. Ann. Surg. *169*, 502 (1969)

Moertel, C.G., Hill, J.R., Adson, M.A.: Surgical management of multiple polyposis. The problem of cancer in the retained bowel segment. Arch. Surg. *100*, 521 (1970)

O'Donnell, W.E., Day, E., Venet, L.: Early detection and diagnosis of cancer. St. Louis: Mosby 1962

Ottenjann, R.: Dickdarmpolypen und koloskopische Polypektomie. Dtsch. Med. Wochenschr. *98*, 677 (1973)

Papaionnon, A., Critselis, A.: Malignant changes in Peutz-Jeghers syndrome. N. Engl. J. Med. *289*, 694 (1973)

Quan, S.H.A., Castro, E.B.: Papillary adenomas (villous tumors): A review of 215 cases. Dis. Colon Rectum *14*, 267 (1971)
Reid, J.D.: Intestinal carcinoma in the Peutz-Jeghers syndrome. J. Am. Med. Assoc. *229*, 833 (1974)
Richardson, J.D.: Villous adenoma: The premalignant dilemma. Am. Surg. *40*, 406 (1974)
Sachatello, C.R.: Familial polyposis of the colon: A four decade follow-up. Cancer *28*, 581 (1971)
Savic, B., Schulz, D., Raschke, E.: Über das Coloncarcinom. Bruns Beitr. Klin. Chir. *219*, 524 (1972)
Shnug, G.E.: Familial polyposis of the colon. Ann. Surg. *37*, 449 (1971)
Vajrabukka, C.: Villous adenoma of rectum. Am. J. Proctol. *24*, 33 (1973)
Velcek, F.T., Coopersmith, I.S., Chen, C.K., Kassner, E.G., Klotz, D.H., Kottmeier, P.K.: Familial juvenile adenomatous polyposis. J. Pediatr. Surg. *11*, 781 (1976)
Watne, A.L., Lai, H.Y., Carrier, J., Coppula, W.: The diagnosis and treatment of patients with Gardner's syndrome. Surgery *82*, 327 (1977)

19 Endometriosis

Occasionally, ectopic islands of uterine endometrium may be seen in the rectal mucosa. The endoscopic appearance is one of circumscribed protrusions that shine with a bluish tint and during menstruation may bleed. Rectal endometriosis can practically never be differentiated from carcinoma grossly. The histologically proven endometriosis should be surgically excised.

References

March, C.M., Israel, R.: Rectovaginal endometriosis: An isolated enigma. Am. J. Obstet. Gynecol. *125*, 274 (1976)
Prexl, H.J., Vilits, P.: Pathogenese, Klinik und Therapie der Dickdarmendometriose. Zentralbl. Chir. *101*, 1112 (1976)
Röher, H.D., Grözinger, K.H.: Zur Klinik, Diagnostik und Therapie der Dickdarmendometriose. Med. Welt *24*, 534 (1973)

20 Pneumatosis Cystoides Intestinalis

(Plate XVI/5 and 6)

Pneumatosis cystoides intestinalis is a condition wherein gas-containing cysts ranging in size from a pinhead to a cherry occur in the wall of the small intestine, the cecum, and the left side of the colon. Involvement of the entire colon has also been reported. The illness can appear at any age. Microscopically with serial sections, one finds a communicating network of gas cysts that are submucosally located in young people and subserosa in older individuals. The composition of the gas is the same as the breath.

Etiologically, the possibility also exists that air may penetrate through small mucosal defects with rectoscopy. Frequently associated with pneumatosis cystoides are other abdominal illnesses such as stomach ulcer and/or carcinoma, pyloric or intestinal stenoses, or a mesenteric tuberculosis. Another hypothesis, supported by animal experiments, suggests that ruptured alveolae with lung diseases permit air to traverse the mediastinum along the vascular sheaths into the wall of the bowel.

Endoscopically, the cysts appear as spheric protrusions in the mucosa and resemble transparent sessile polyps. Biopsy permits the air in the cysts to escape so that they collapse. The diagnosis is most often made radiologically with air-contrast barium examination. The bubbles outline the wall of the bowel like pearls on a string.

The clinical symptoms found with pneumatosis cystoides resemble those of an irritable bowel: nonspecific abdominal spasms with constipation, rarely diarrhea with blood or mucus. Pneumoperitoneum as a complication may occur when the cysts rupture. Treatment is necessary only when diarrhea containig blood and mucous is present, and in these cases a nonabsorbable antibiotic or bismuth preparation may be helpful or hyperbaric oxygin may be used. Symptoms similar to irritable bowel should otherwise be treated symptomatically. Resection of the bowel is only indicated for the treatment of occlusion or infection.

References

Culver, G.J.: Pneumatosis intestinalis with associated retroperitoneal air. Report of a complication of severe asthma. J. Am. Med. Assoc. *186*, 160 (1963)

De Jong, R.H.: Gas in the gut wall. J. Am. Med. Assoc. *237*, 1965 (1977)

Forde, K.A., Whitelock, R.T., Seaman, W.B.: Pneumatosis and cystoides intestinalis. Report of a case with colonoscopic findings of inflammatory bowel disease. Am. J. Gastroenterol. *68*, 188 (1977)

Goodall, R.J.: Pneumatosis coli: Report of two cases. Dis. Colon Rectum *21*, 61 (1978)

Masterson, J.S., Fratkin, L.B., Osler, T.R., Trapp, W.G.: Treatment of pneumatosis cystoides intestinalis with hyperbaric oxygen. Am. Surg. *183*, 245 (1978)

Varano, V.J., Bonanno, C.A.: Colonoscopic findings in pneumatosis cystoides intestinalis. Am. J. Gastroenterol. *59*, 353 (1973)

Wertkin, M.G., Wetchler, B.B., Waye, J.D., Brown, L.K.: Pneumatosis coli associated with sigmoid volvulus and colonoscopy. Am. J. Gastroenterol. *65*, 209 (1976)

Yale, C.E., Balish, E.: Pneumatosis cystoides intestinalis. Dis. Colon Rectum *19*, 107 (1976)

21 Solitary Rectal Ulcer

(Plate XIX/1)

Solitary ulcers of the rectum may be traumatic in origin and caused by thermometers, occasionally by digital removal of a fecal impaction, or by deviate sexual behavior. Solitary rectal ulcers may also be a manifestation of Crohn's disease. Very rarely, ectopic gastric mucosa is their cause. For the vast majority of solitary rectal ulcers, the explanation remains unknown. Occasionally, the ulcers are accompanied by localized inflammation of the mucosa within the distal segment of the rectum with edema, erythema, and circumscribed whitish flecks in a thickened bowel wall covered by excessive secretions. The changes are found predominantly in the ventral portion of the rectum, and in contrast to the adjacent normal mucosa are strikingly apparent. *Neiger* refers to these changes as a proctitis terminalis simplex. Local injury, such as locally administered medication or local irritation of the mucosa, has been proposed as an etiologic factor. Conjecturally, mechanical alterations through strangulation of prolapsed areas of mucosa with compromise of the arterial blood supply in cases of chronic constipation and straining at the stool during defecation may also play a role.

Not infrequently the chronic bleeding and induration here is confused with carcinoma, with the result that the rectum is surgically removed. The assurance gained from adequate tissue sampling by biopsy is therefore of great value in these cases. If a carcinoma cannot be unequivocally diagnosed, surgery need not be performed for the removal of a solitary rectal ulcer.

References

Cox, R.W.: A case of gastric heterotopia in the rectum. J. Pathol. Bacteriol. *84*, 427 (1962)

Gordon, B.S., Clyman, D.: Barium granuloma of the rectum. Gastroenterology *32*, 943 (1957)

Madigan, M.R., Morson, B.C.: Solitary ulcer of the rectum. J. Br. Soc. Gastroenterol. *10*, 871 (1969)

Neiger, A.: Proctitis terminalis simplex. Z. Gastroenterol. *7*, 694 (1976)

Riek, M., Halter, F., Stirnemann, H.: Das solitäre Rektalulkus. Schweiz. Med. Wochenschr. *101*, 758 (1971)

22 Anastomoses (Ileorectal; Colorectal)

(Plates XIV/1 and XIX/4)

With disease processes that involve the large bowel but leave the rectum free (Crohn's disease, diverticulitis, neoplasms), a surgical procedure used for their treatment will result in an anastomosis that may be seen during rectoscopy. During the postoperative follow-up period, careful attention should be given to any recurrence, which in cases of Crohn's disease is seen very early on rectoscopy.

23 Fistulae (Rectovaginal, Rectovesical)

(Plate XIX/2)

The clinical manifestations of a fistula – stool from the vagina, air from the urethra – are often difficult to recognize because the fistulous opening is hidden by the edematous and swollen mucosa. Larger defects occur particularly after radiation therapy and with Crohn's disease.

24 Ureteral Transplantation

In cases of obstruction of the bladder and urethra that cannot be corrected surgically, the ureters are transplanted into the rectum or sigma. These may be visualized during rectoscopy. They appear as small erections that, with the intravenous injection of a dye such as methylene blue or phenol red, become more obvious as the dye is eliminated in the urine.

25 Melena (Plate XIX/5)

When the patient states that blood has been passed in the stool, a rectoscopic clarification of the source for the bleeding is necessary. Melena indicates a bleeding site in the upper gastrointestinal tract above the cecum, while bleeding from lower down leads to the passage of fresh or coagulated blood. It is also possible that such bleeding may arise from the hemorrhoidal area (e.g., thermometer injuries) and having flowed cephalad while the patient has been lying down and been acted upon by colon bacteria appears only the next day as a tarry stool.

26 Foreign Bodies

Various forms of undigested food such as peelings from fruits, vegetables, salads, fruit kernels, etc. can be seen during rectoscopy. Foreign bodies that have been swallowed can traverse the entire gastrointestinal tract and become lodged at the internal anal sphincter. They can be then removed with the rectoscope.

Plates I–XIX

Plate I/1–6

1 Capillary network in the rectal ampulla. The delicately branched vessels constitute an important endoscopic criterion for a normal mucosa.

2 Increased filling of the vessels. The degree of filling of these vessels in the mucosa shows extensive functional variation and is influenced by psychological factors, mucosa irritation by enema, etc. An increased degree of filling in these vessels and reddening of the mucosa is not of any clinical significance as long as the branching of the small vessels is clearly visible. This should therefore not be considered a "mild form of colitis."

Factitial Lesions

3 Factitial bleeding. The punctate bleeding areas in the mucosa are abrasions caused by the passage of the rectoscope through a curve in the colon.

4 Factitial erosions. In the center, an erosion behind a fold of Morgagni on the ventral wall of the bowel can be seen. This area lies in a straight extension of the anal canal. The erosion was caused by a temperature thermometer. The symptom that led to the examination was melena. During the night, after the evening temperature measurement had been taken, the rectal ampulla filled with blood. The blood underwent change from fresh to tarry in nature.

5 Factitial ulcer. The ulcer was caused by the unprofessional introduction of the enema tip. This was an incidental diagnosis without symptoms.

6 Condition after suction biopsy of the superficial mucosa without significant bleeding: lentil-sized defect in the mucosa.

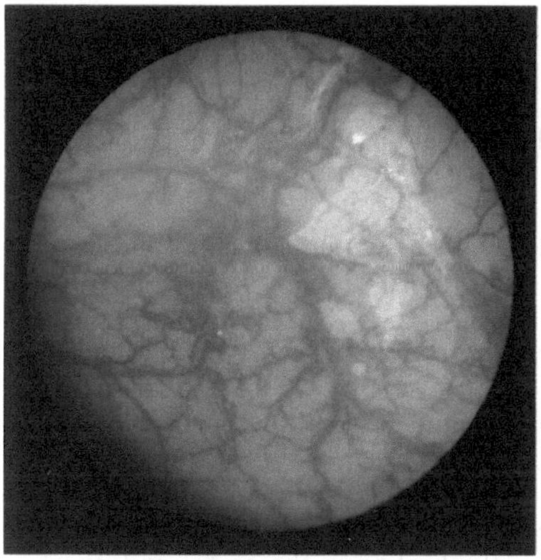
1

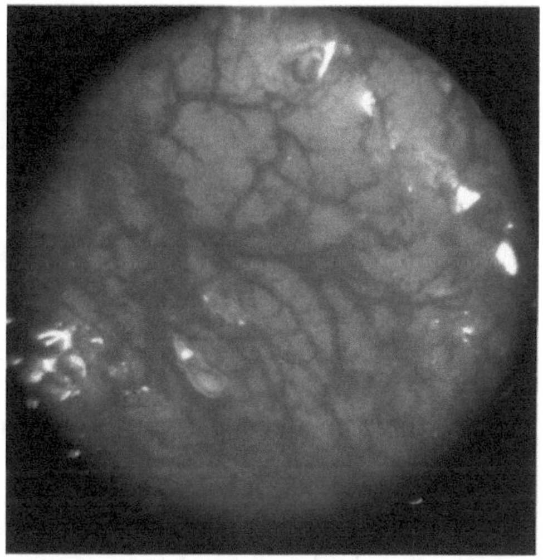
2

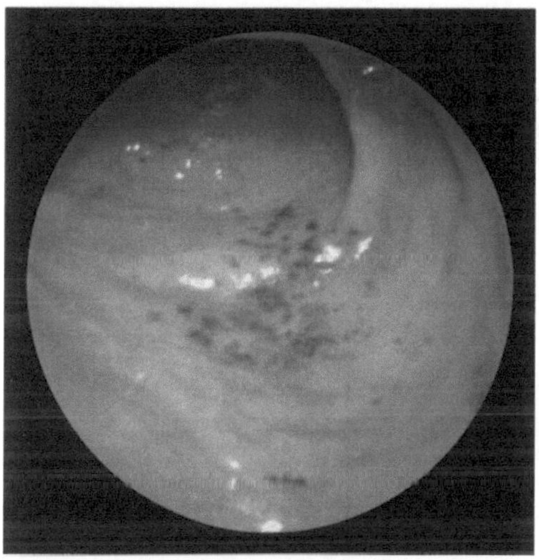
3

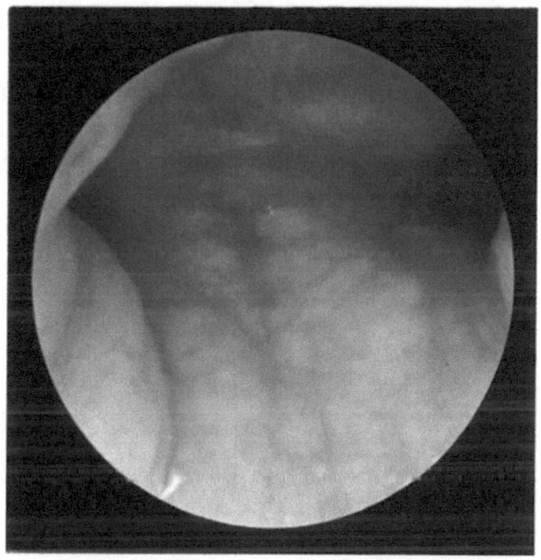
4

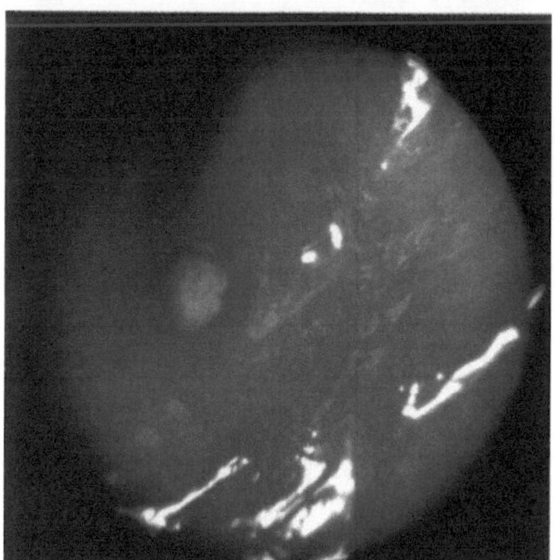
5

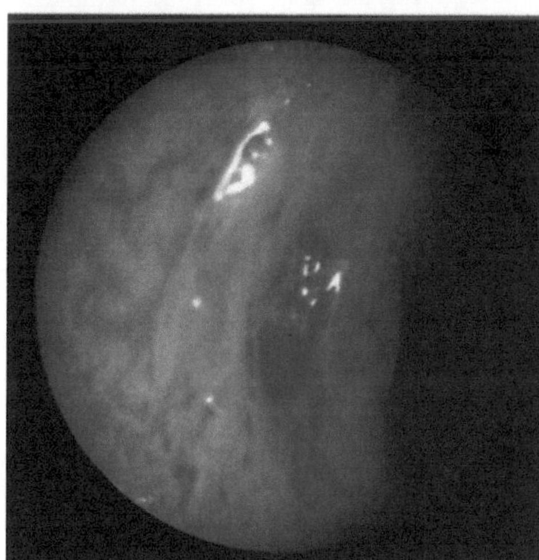
6

Plate II/1–6

1 Melanosis recti. Leopard-skin mucosal demarcation as the result of chronic laxative abuse with plant laxatives.

2 Melanosis recti. Dark discoloration of the mucosa with the lymph follicles appearing whitish.

3 Acute perianal eczema with prominent erythema and some maceration.

4 Chronic anal eczema with marked pruritis and whitish thickening of the anal skin (lichenification).

5 Chronic anal eczema with superimposed mycotic infection with spreading to the cheeks. Typical for a mycosis is the healing in the center and an accentuated border.

6 Hemorrhoidal tags. A common harmless finding of variable size occurring, for instance, as the result of a previous perianal thrombosis. Hemorrhoidal tags do not fill up with abdominal pressure and are thereby distinguished from external hemorrhoids.

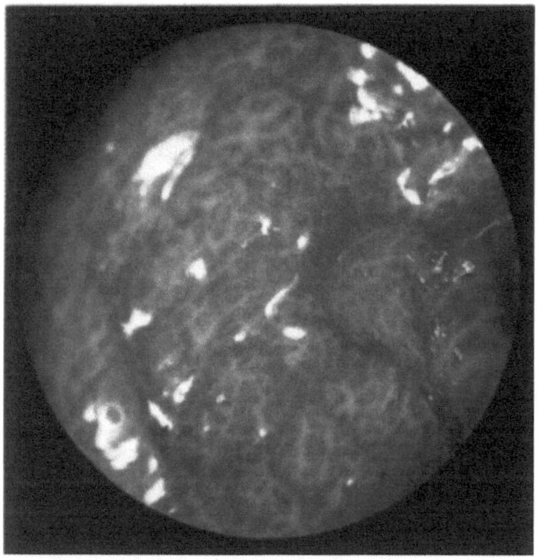
1

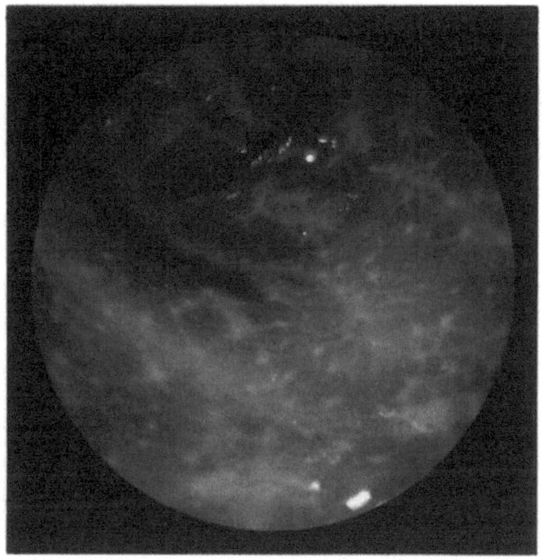
2

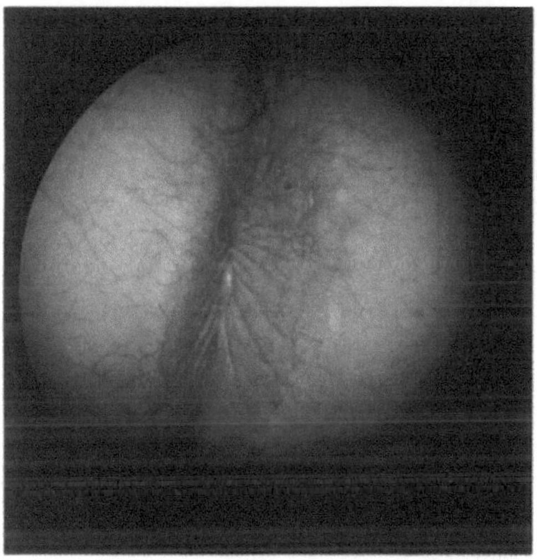
3

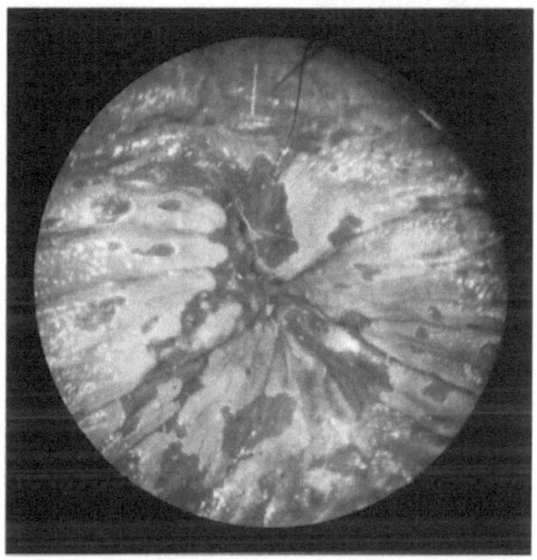
4

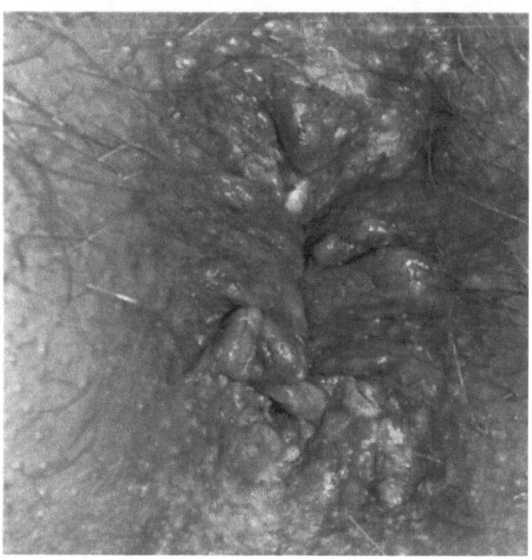
5

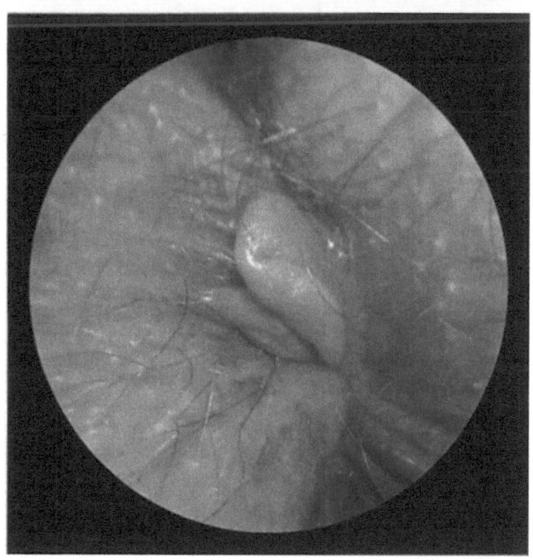
6

Plate III/1–6

1 Cherry-sized, bluish perianal thrombosis at 6:00 o'clock, which has suddenly appeared and caused extreme discomfort. The hemorrhoidal tag at 12:00 o'clock is an incidental finding.

2 Puncture incision of a perianal thrombosis using the pointed scalpel without prior anesthesia.

3 Under slight pressure, the thrombus is extruded and the patient becomes symptom-free.

4 Perianal thrombosis after spontaneous perforation. The discomfort subsides but bleeding may persist for days. With slight pressure, the thrombus may be expressed.

5 External hemorrhoids, not filled, not painful, soft knots covered with normal squamous epithelium.

6 The same external hemorrhoids as in Plate III/5 after abdominal pressure. The knots fill tightly but are elastic and can be evacuated by the finger.

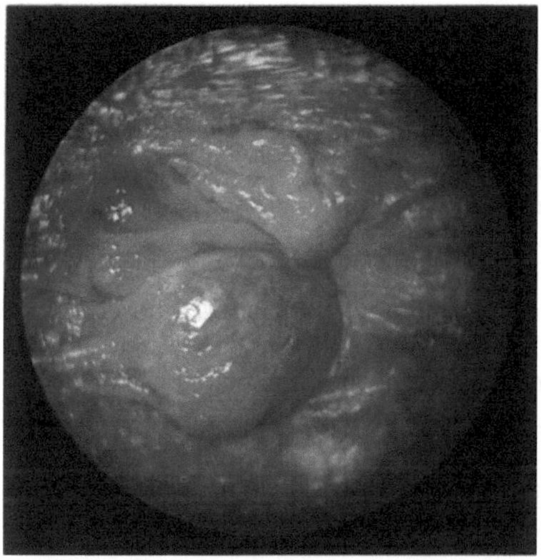

1

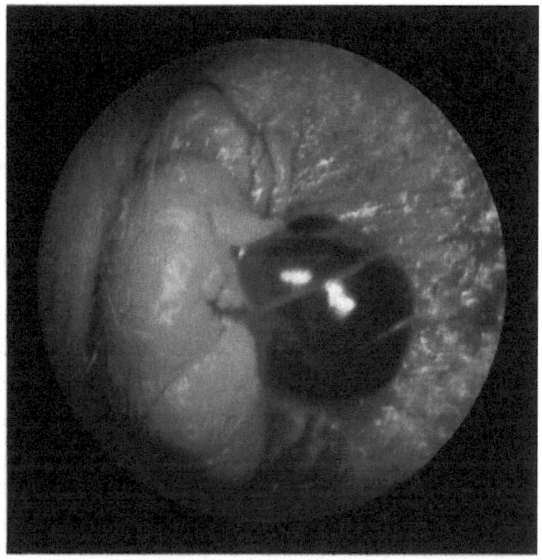

2

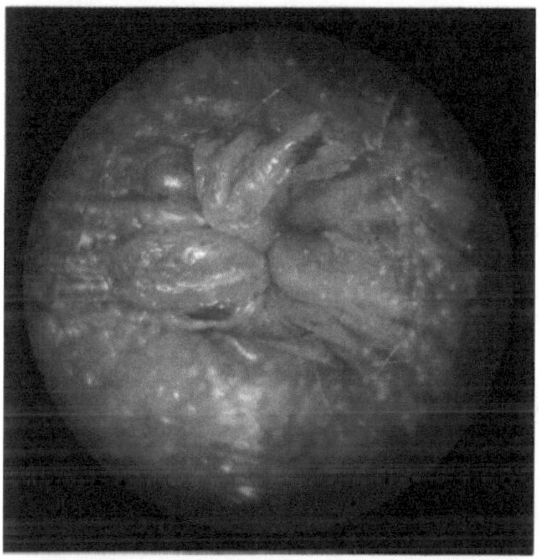

3

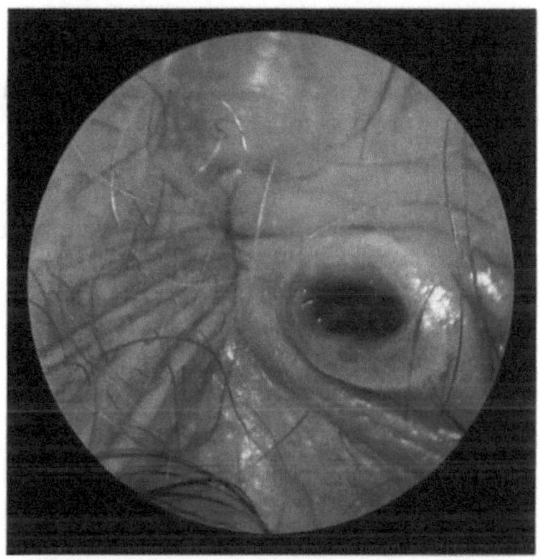

4

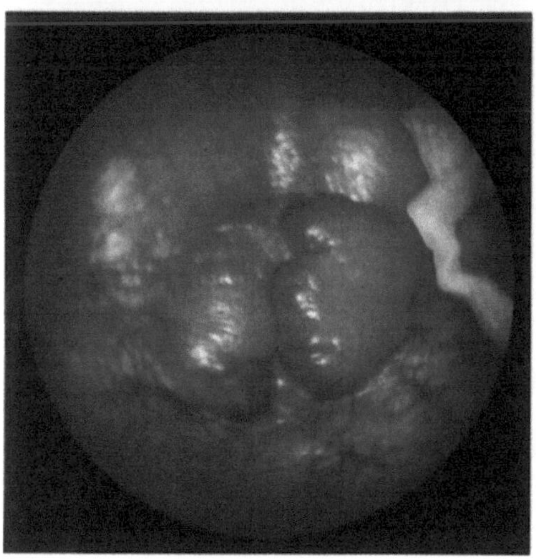

5

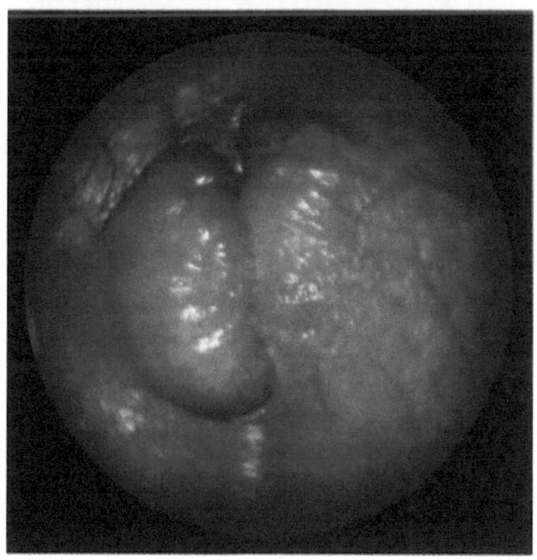

6

Plate IV/1–6

1 Acute anal fissure. Long, oval ulcer in the typical location at the posterior commissure (12:00 o'clock in knee-chest position) with greyish-yellow, dirty base. Because of severe pain, the examination was done under local anesthesia.

2 Chronic anal fissure, 6 weeks old, with undermined, light calloused border. A typical sentinel fold indicates the location of the fissure. The base of the fissure has been cleaned. Often one can see in the base of the chronic fissure the transverse fibers of the internal anal sphincter.

3 Pointed condylomata (condylomata acuminata), wart-like, arranged like blades of grass, small tumors of sandy-colored appearance.

4 Pointed condylomata extending into the anal canal.

5 Broad condylomata (condylomata lata), moist, wide-based papules in contrast to the finger-like, pointed condylomata.

6 Broad condylomata (condylomata lata), broad-based papules at the anterior commissure in a case of secondary lues.

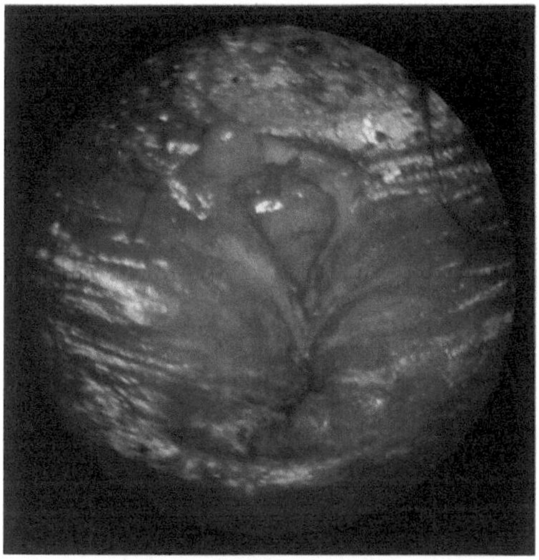

1

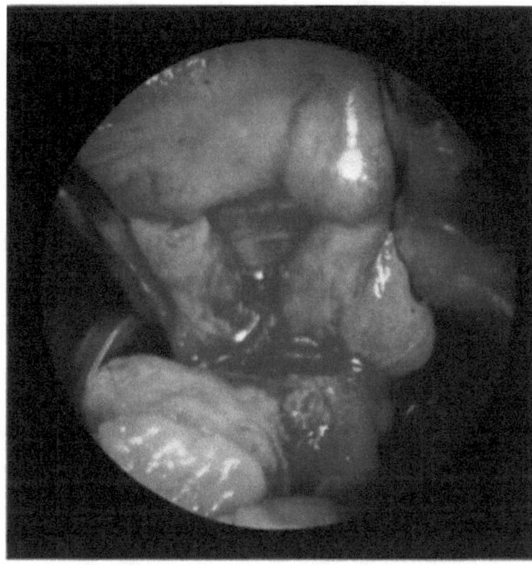

2

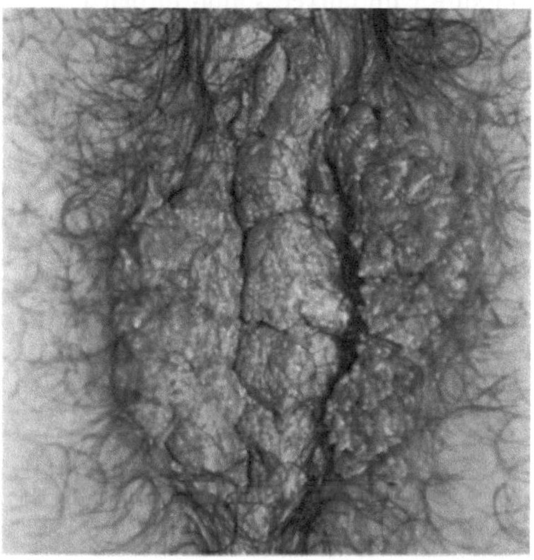

3

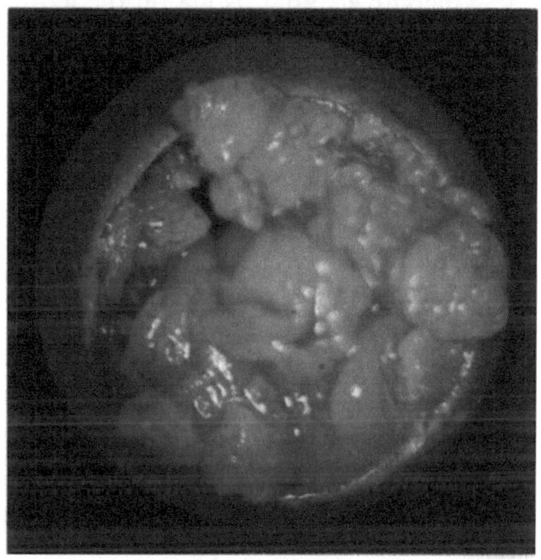

4

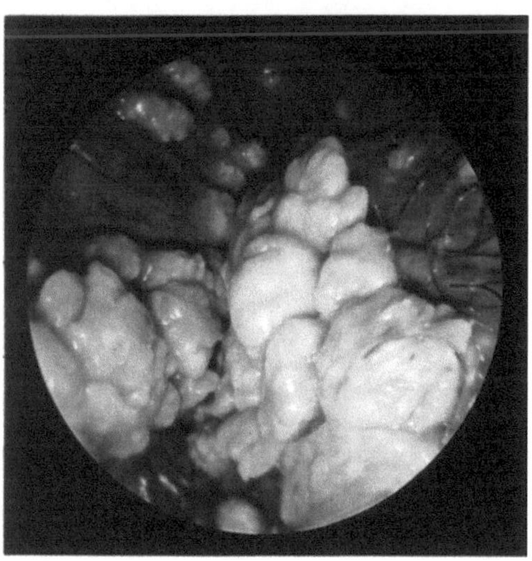

5

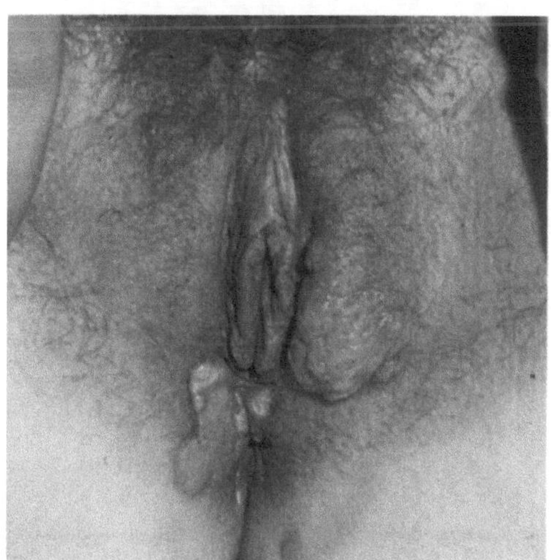

6

Plate V/1–6

1 Anal fistula with button sound in tract.

2 The button sound containing a nonabsorbable suture has been placed through the fistulous tract.

3 Severe perianal fistulae with the formation of a horseshoe fistulous tract as a complication of Crohn's disease.

4 Horseshoe fistula with thread drainage; under this treatment, the perianal infiltration has regressed leaving widespread asymptomatic secondary fistulous openings.

5 Incomplete anal fistula on the left commissure with curved sound in place.

6 Entrance of an incomplete internal fistula with inlaid curved sound demonstrated through an anal speculum. Such changes can only be evaluated with the help of an anal speculum.

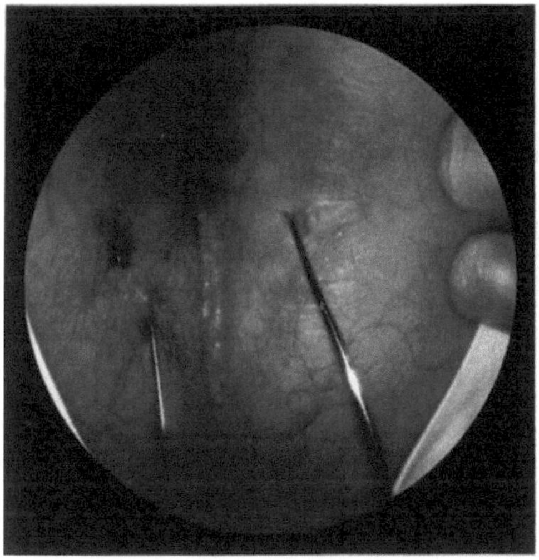
1

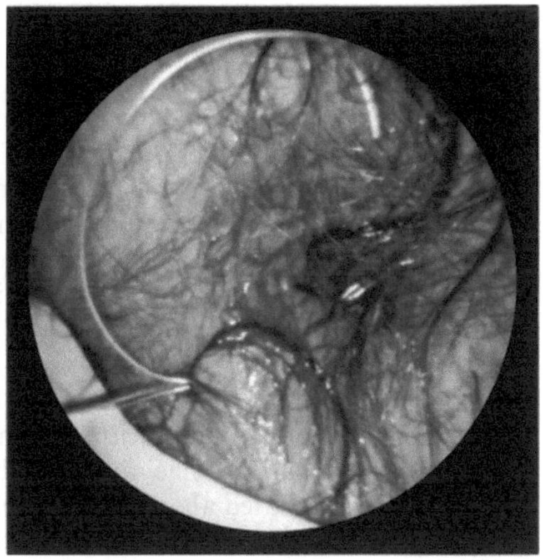
2

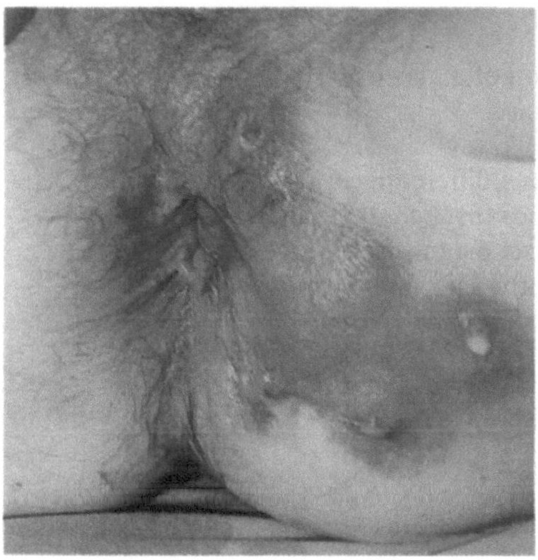
3

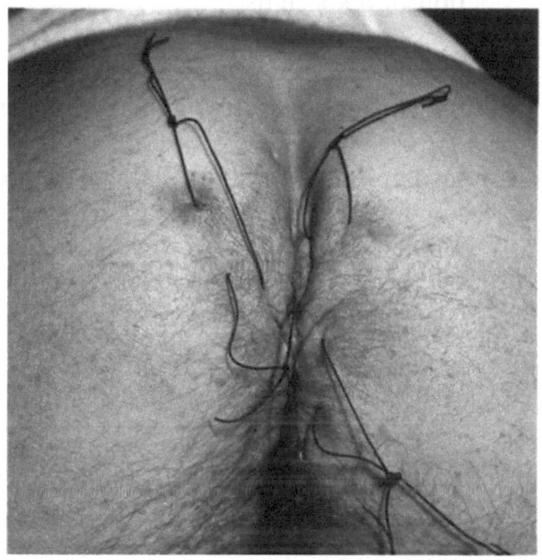
4

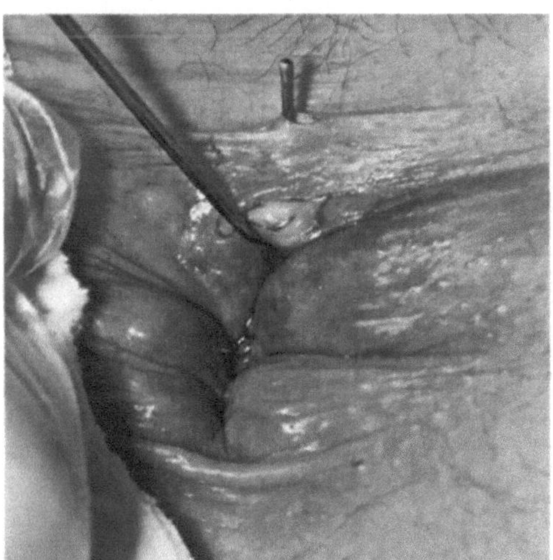
5

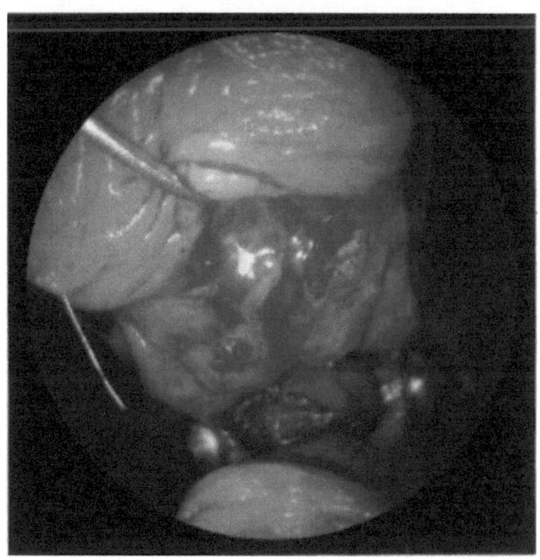
6

Plate VI/1–4

1 Secondary anal prolapse, end stage of hemorrhoidal disease, stage III hemorrhoids, with knots around the anal margin that are reducible and covered with mucosa in contrast to prolapsing anal fibromas, hemorrhoidal tags, or carcinoma of the anus. The mucosa protrudes as a bulge or a knot and has been altered by inflammation. Not infrequently the prolapsing knots are lividly colored, elastic, and especially apparent after strangulation by the sphincter ani.

2 Carcinoma of the anus with minimal symptoms and slow growth in a 75-year-old patient. The similarity between this carcinoma and the anal prolapse illustrated above makes it understandable that the carcinoma was diagnosed 9 months after the first examination and only then by consultation of a specialist.

3 Complete rectal prolapse with protrusion of all layers of the bowel, circular fold formation, and telescopic appearance.

4 Carcinoma of the anus that can be grossly differentiated from hemorrhoidal tags and prolapsing stage III hemorrhoids through its firmness on palpation and its very irregular surface. For an exact diagnosis, histologic examination of biopsy tissue is necessary. Frequently this finding is misdiagnosed as "hemorrhoids," as was the case in this patient.

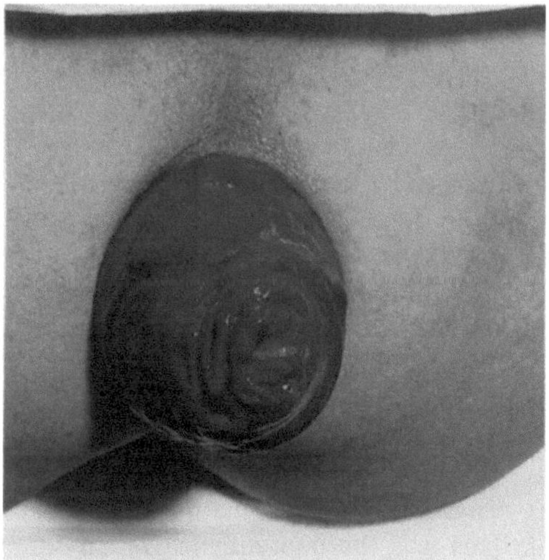

1

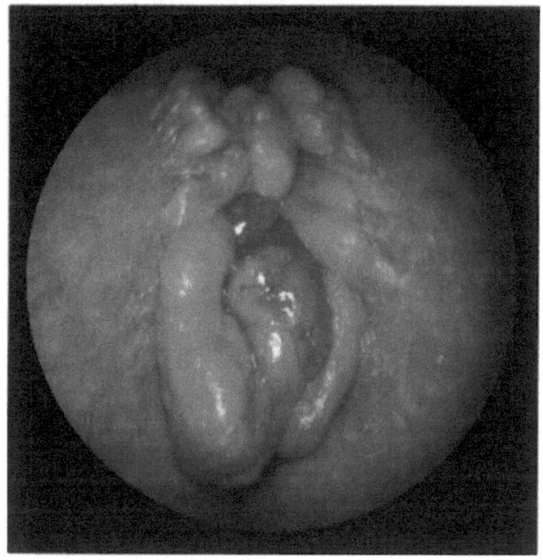

2

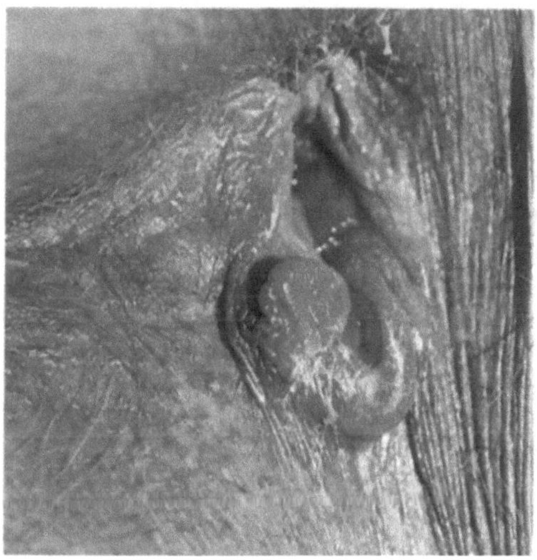

3

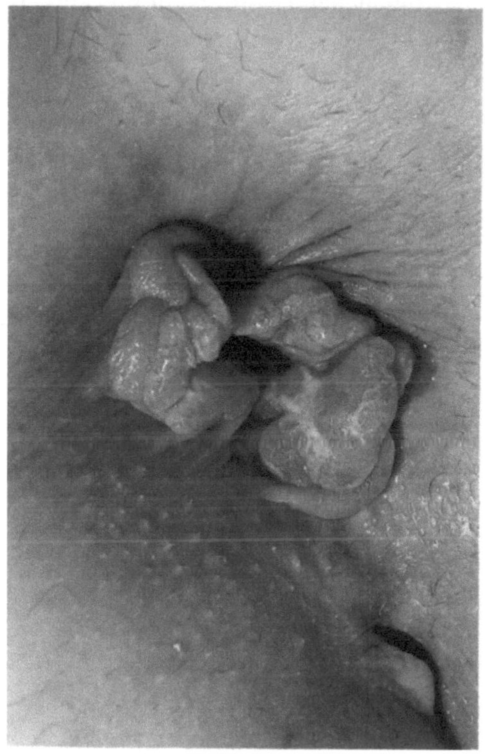

4

Plate VII/1–6

1 Purulent anitis in a case of lues. Pus empties from the anal canal. At 10:00 o'clock condylomata lata may be seen. The picture was taken in a prostitute who because of severe discomfort in the anal region sought medical care. The first thought was a fresh anal fissure.

2 Acute cryptitis and proctitis. In the foreground are the whitish papillae of Morgagni. The folds of Morgagni with the crypts lying in between are diffusely red. The patient complained about pressure in the anus with wetness and itching.

3 Hypertrophied anal papillae (cat's tooth). A hypertrophied papilla protrudes from the right side into the anal canal. This was the consequence of an inflammatory process in this area. In contrast to soft spongy hemorrhoids, this can be felt during digital rectal examination.

4 Anal fibroma. Two fibromas have prolapsed outward.

5 Floating anal fibroma. From above, a pedunculated whitish object hangs into the anal canal. This anal fibroma constitutes an advanced stage of hypertrophy of an anal papilla. The anal fibroma is not a neoplasm and has no malignant potential.

6 The fibroma has prolapsed through the anal canal. During the bowel movement, it may protrude outward, be unable to return because of the anal sphincter, and then cause discomfort.

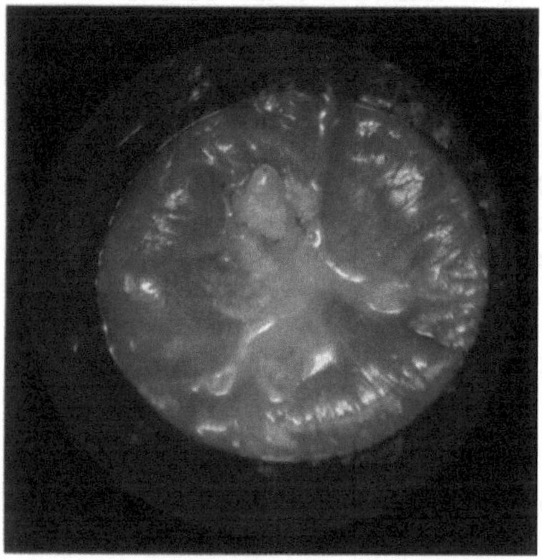
1

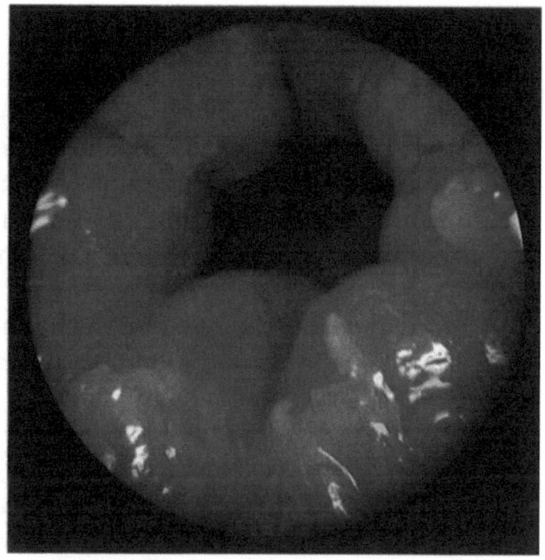
2

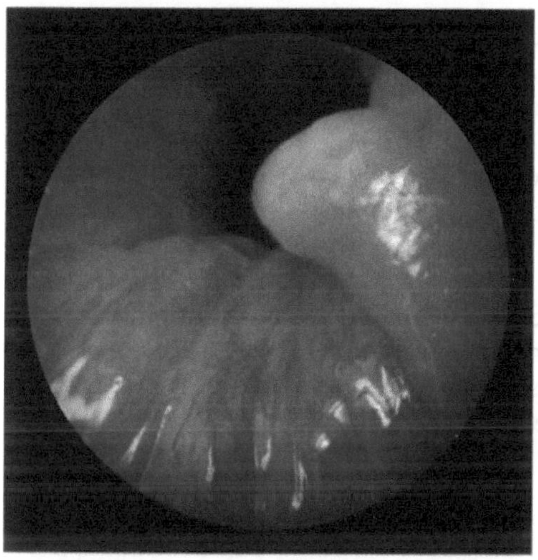
3

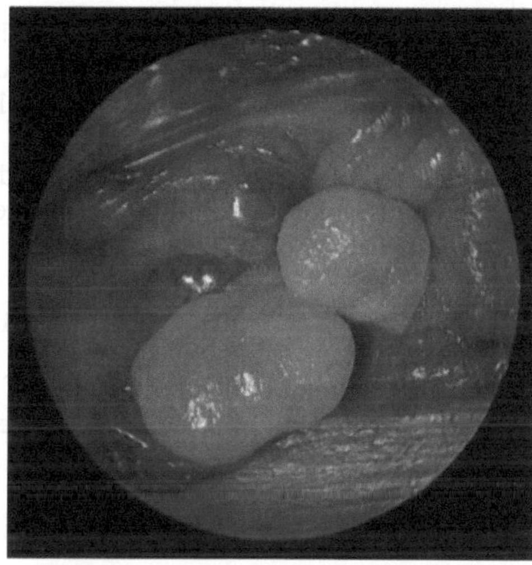
4

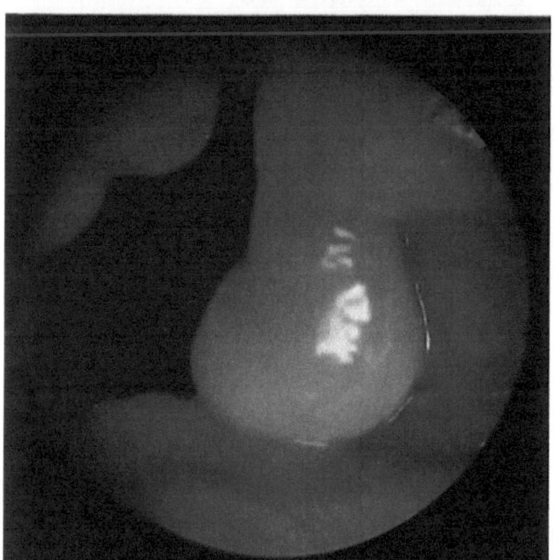
5

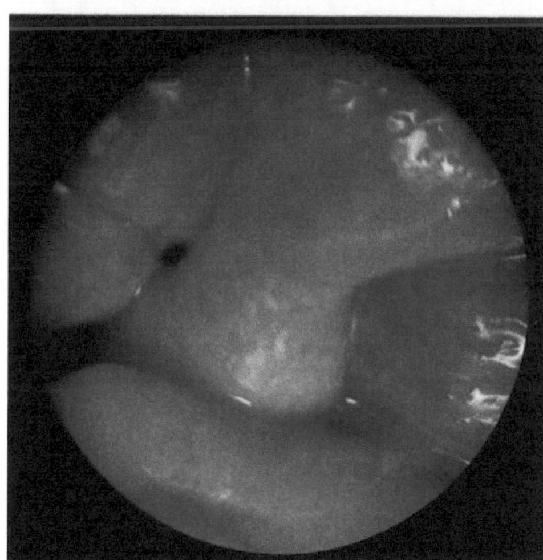
6

Plate VIII/1–6

1 Stage I hemorrhoids. The hemorrhoidal knots protrude into the endoscope without, however, prolapsing. At 2:00 and 10:00 o'clock, reddish areas are recognizable that indicate superficial defects in the overlying mucosa from which the hemorrhoidal bleeding arises.

2 Stage II hemorrhoids. The hemorrhoidal knots prolapsed some distance into the endoscope. Following defecation, they protruded out of the anus but retracted spontaneously.

3 Stage III hemorrhoids (anal prolapse). The hemorrhoids prolapsed outward and did not retract. The reddish mucous membrane covering shows up against the surrounding hemorrhoidal tags.

4 Grade I hemorrhoids. The hemorrhoids protrude into the proctoscope through the side window. The superficial mucosa also shows slight bleeding. In the rear, a mirrow showing the other side of the hemorrhoid.

5 Hemorrhoid sclerosing. Using a needle that is angulated at 45°, 0.1–0.3 ml of a 20% quinine solution are injected strictly submucosally into the base of the hemorrhoid.

6 Injection ulcer. With a superficial injection of the sclerosing solution, the mucosa turns red and ulcerates. This may be misinterpreted as a carcinoma if one is not aware of its cause. If such an ulcer develops in a patient with a coagulation defect, serious bleeding may occur.

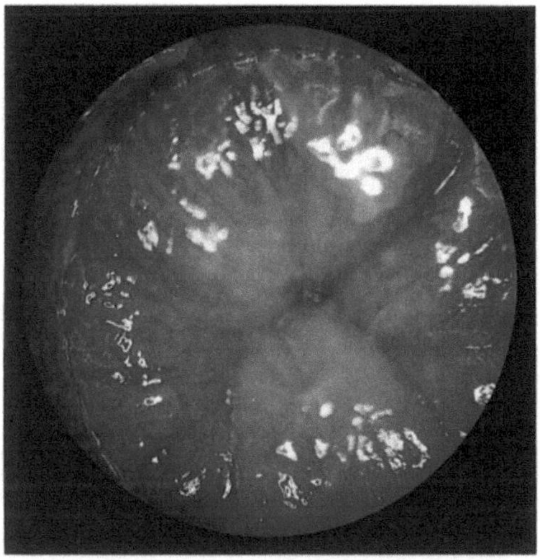

1

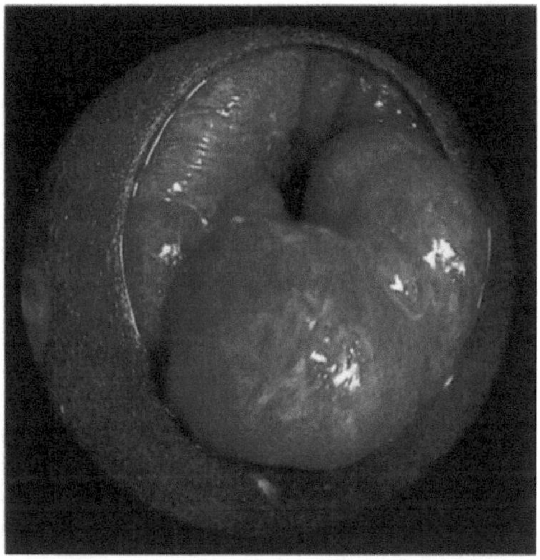

2

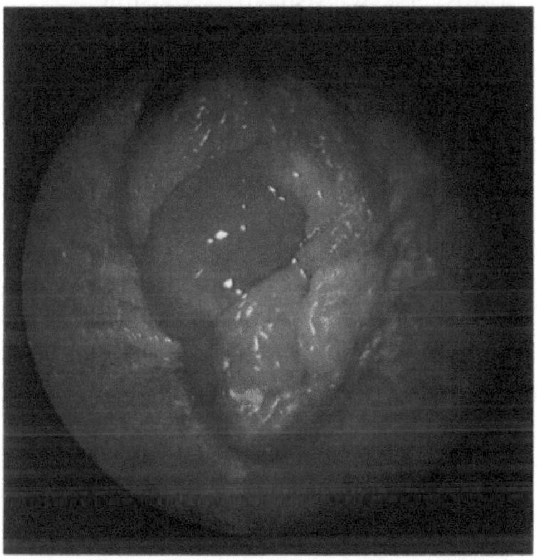

3

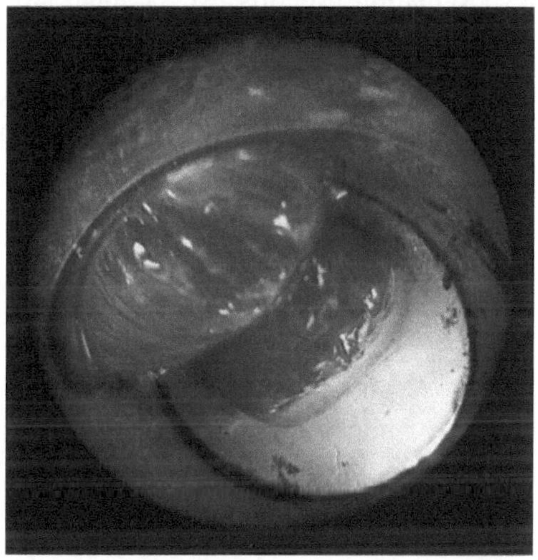

4

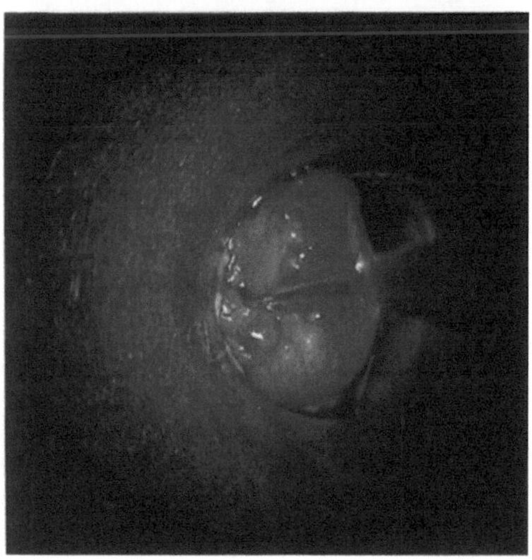

5

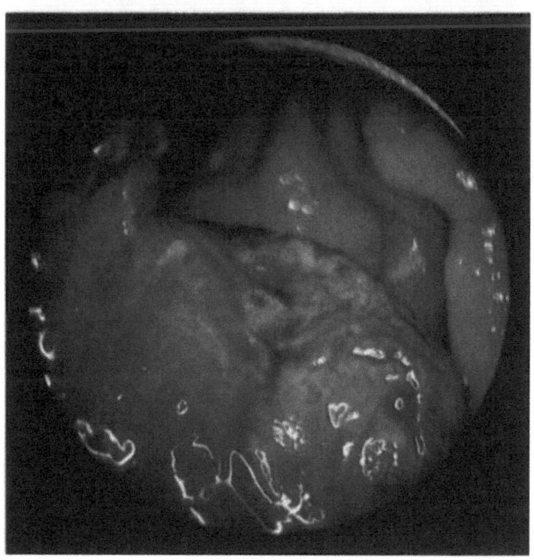

6

Plate IX/1–6

1 Proctitis associated with an ischiorectal abscess. The mucosa is edematous and the vascular pattern is absent. A longitudinal fold protrudes from below into the bowel lumen. Dull pain was present in the anal region. No abnormal findings were detected externally.

2 With biopsy of this fold, pus exuded and the abscess drained through the rectum to the outside.

3 Cryptitis-proctitis. With inflammatory changes in the anal area, the lower portion of the rectum may also become involved and manifest, as in this case, a diffuse redness.

4 Radiation proctitis. At the 8-cm level, a transverse whitish area is visible. The surrounding tissue bleeds with only slight irritation. The patient had noted intermittent rectal bleeding for over 1 year after receiving radiation treatment for a genital carcinoma. The bleeding had become more severe. Histology: Fibrosis and vasculitis without evidence of malignancy.

5 Radiation proctitis. In the foreground obvious necrosis and in the surrounding areas freshly inflamed mucosa can be seen. Above the 10-cm level, a stenosis is present. This condition arose after radiation therapy was given as treatment for a bladder carcinoma. Because of increased pain and the stenosis, a bypass operation was necessary. On histologic examination of the rectal biopsy, no evidence for malignancy was found.

6 Radiation proctitis. This is a late stage of radiation proctitis in which only a bleeding tendency remained.

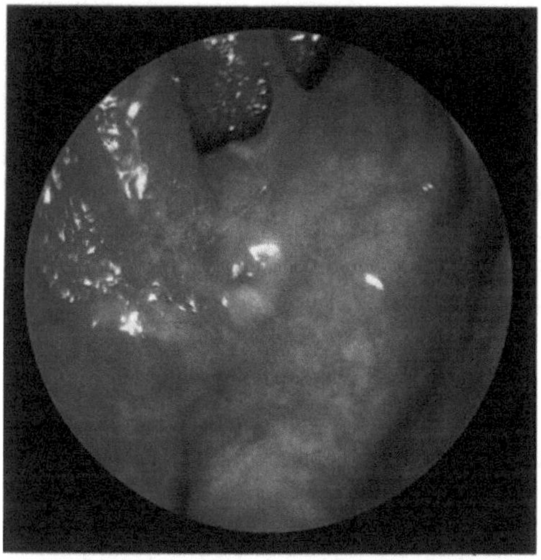
1

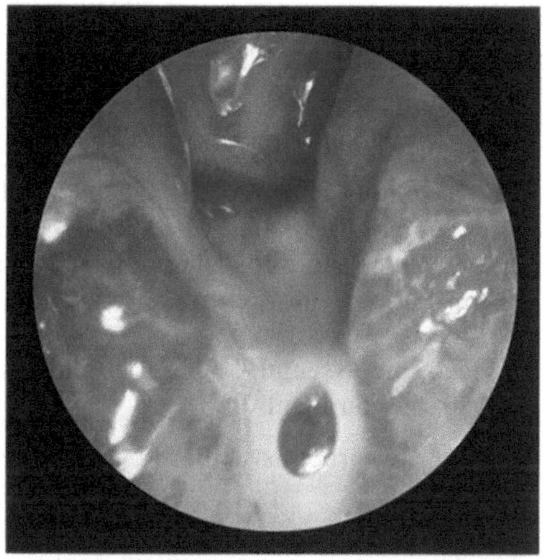
2

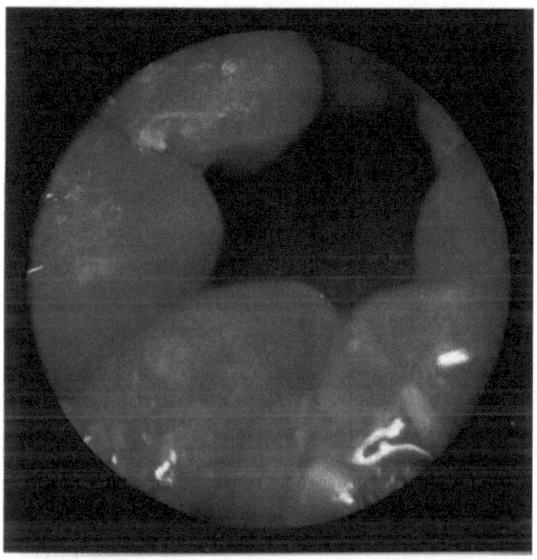
3

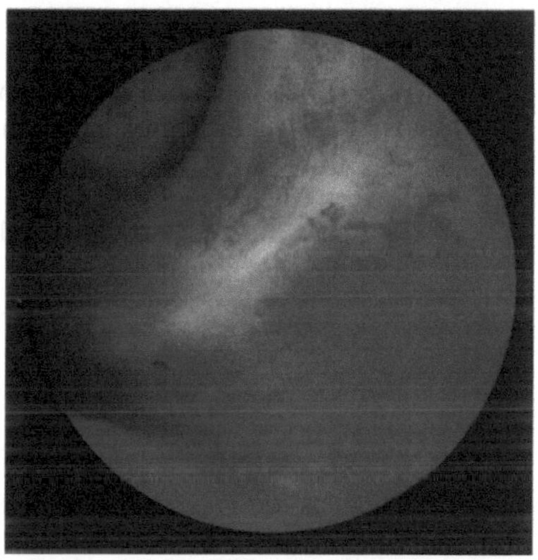
4

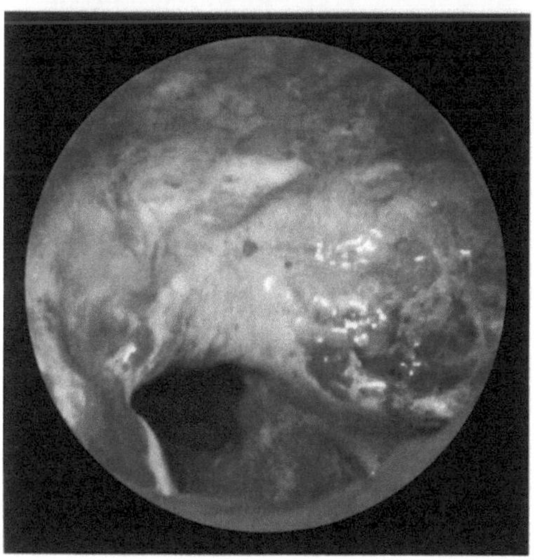
5

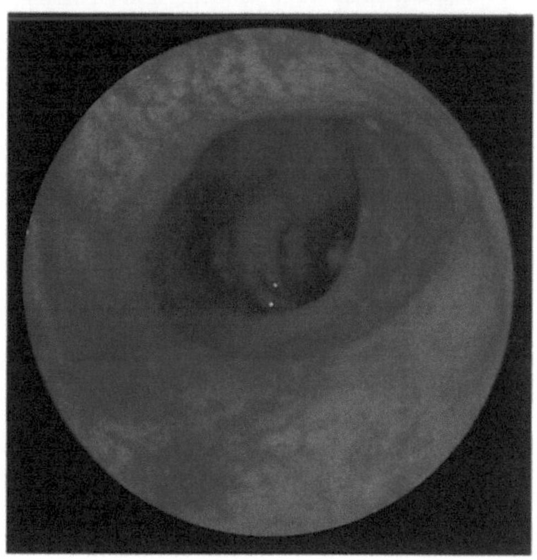
6

Plate X/1–6

Infectious Proctitis

1 Infectious enterocolitis. There are localized bleeding areas with loss of the vascular pattern. A specific cause could not be determined. After 5 days, the acute episode of diarrhea resolved itself without specific treatment and the mucosa returned to a normal appearance.

Amebic dysentary. A tourist had just returned from Persia and developed bloody purulent diarrhea:

2 Diffuse proctitis with absence of the vascular pattern. The mucosa bleeds easily.

3 The mucosa has a purulent coating in which ameba can be demonstrated (*arrows*).

4/5 In the upper rectum there are circumscribed punctate abscesses in association with a generalized inflammation.

6 Ameboma. The patient was operated on for a suspected carcinoma. Biopsy of the tumor showed, however, only inflammation. Ameba were found in the tumor, an "ameboma."

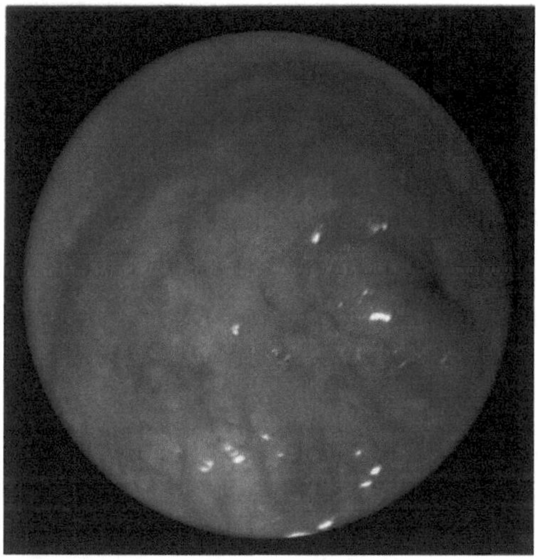

1

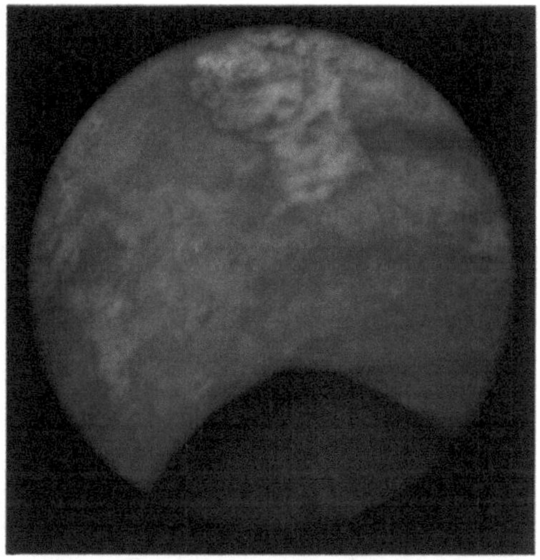

2

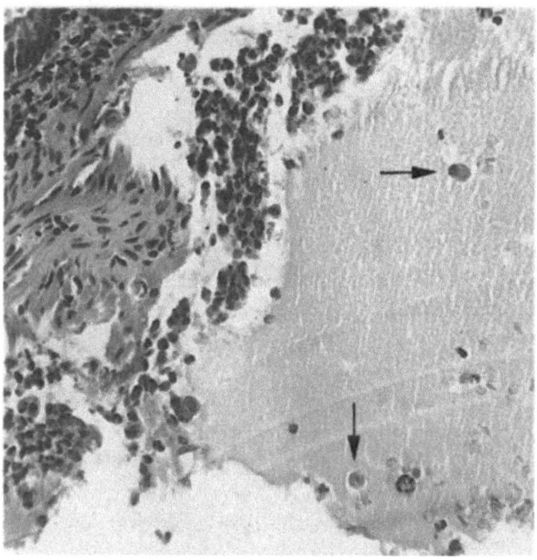

3

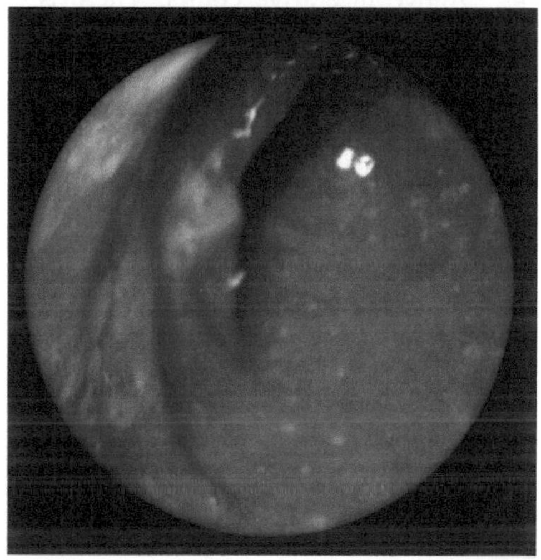

4

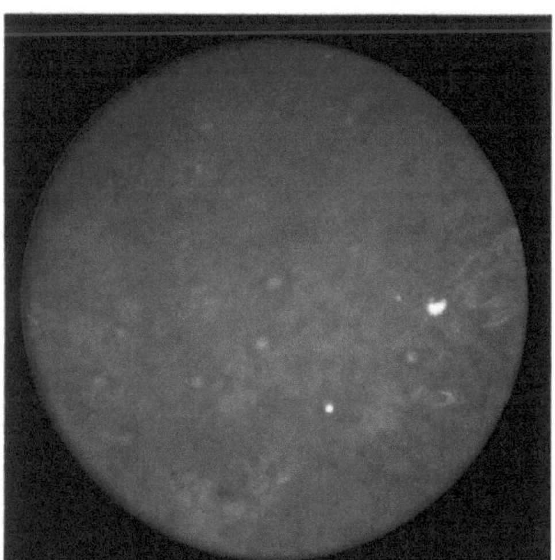

5

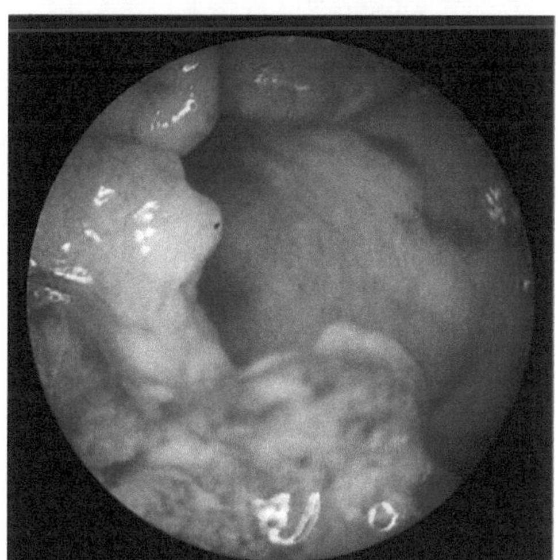

6

Plate XI/1–6

1 Hemorrhagic "ulcerative" proctitis. At the 9-cm level, one finds an abrupt transition from the changes of colitis in the mucosa with increased friability, redness, and edema to an unremarkable mucosa with normal vascular markings. This represents a mild form of ulcerative colitis.

2 Active ulcerative colitis in the acute stage. The mucosal surface is granular and dusty-red. In this and the following cases, a bloody purulent diarrhea was the predominant symptom.

3 Active ulcerative colitis. The folds of Houston in the foreground are edematous and swollen with a purulent lining.

4 Active ulcerative colitis. There is an increased friability in the mucosa, which in this case manifested many punctate bleeding points when touched by the sponge.

5 Active ulcerative colitis. The bleeding on contact is in this case more pronounced.

6 Chronic ulcerative colitis. The mucosa is paler than in the previous case. The vascular pattern is absent and a mucopurulent lining is visible.

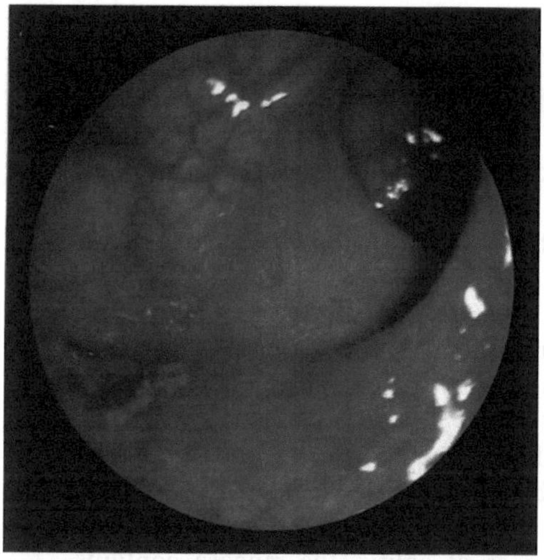

1

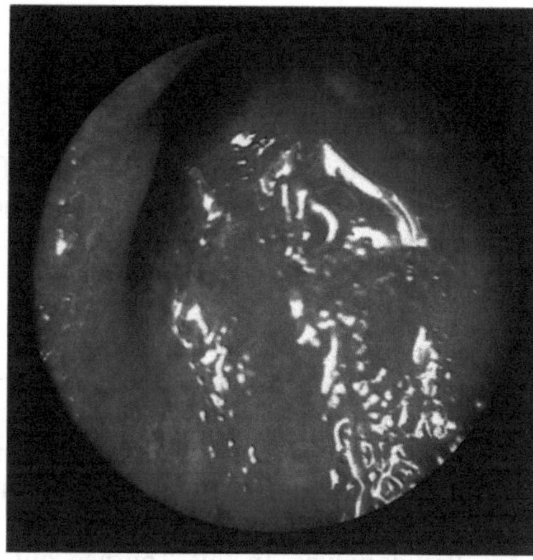

2

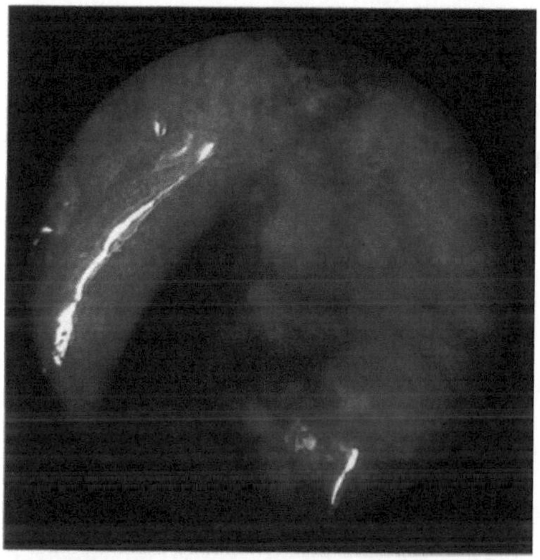

3

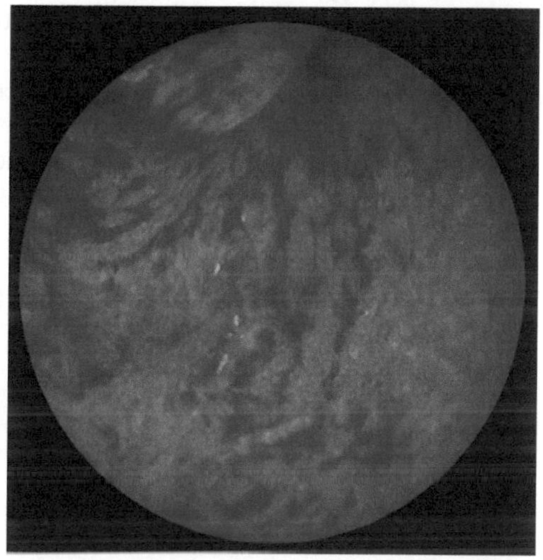

4

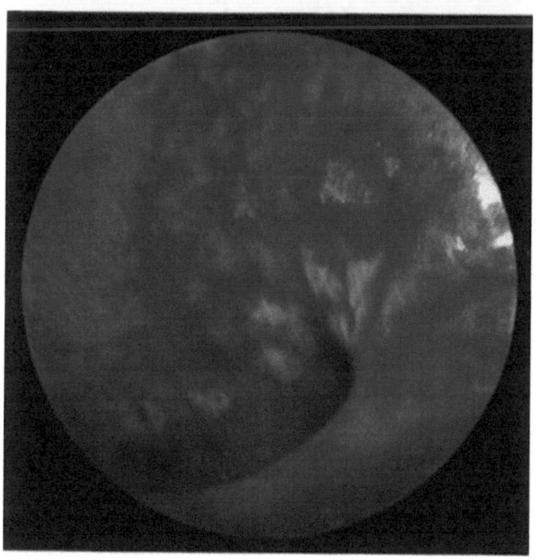

5

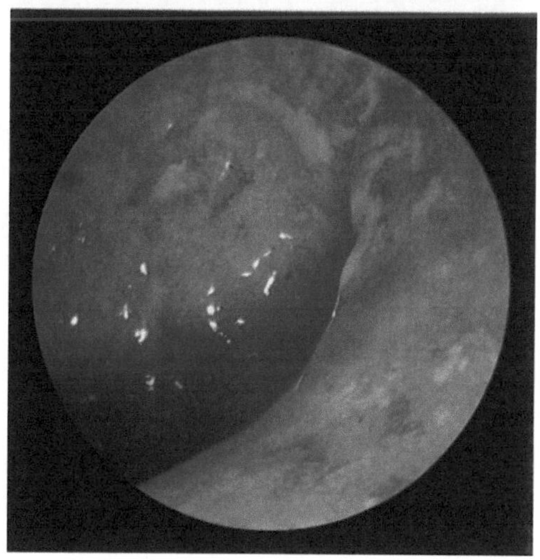

6

Plate XII/1–6

1 Chronic ulcerative colitis in an early stage of remission. The active stage responded to treatment using Azulfidine and prednisone. The increased friability of the mucosa remains. The vascular pattern is still absent. The patient was symptom-free and the stool was formed. Passage of blood and pus was no longer observed.

2 Ulcerative colitis in remission. The normal vascular pattern is partially visible although the mucosa continues to show patchy changes.

3 Pseudopolyps. Large and small islands of mucosa project into the bowel lumen. They are partially covered with pus.

4 Pseudopolyps. In this "burned out" case of colitis, the mucosa contains islands of mucosa (pseudopolyps) intermingled with atrophic areas.

5 Pseudopolyp in a case of ulcerative colitis with exacerbation.

6 Proctitis terminalis simplex with thickened edematous mucosa, increased redness, and ulceration.

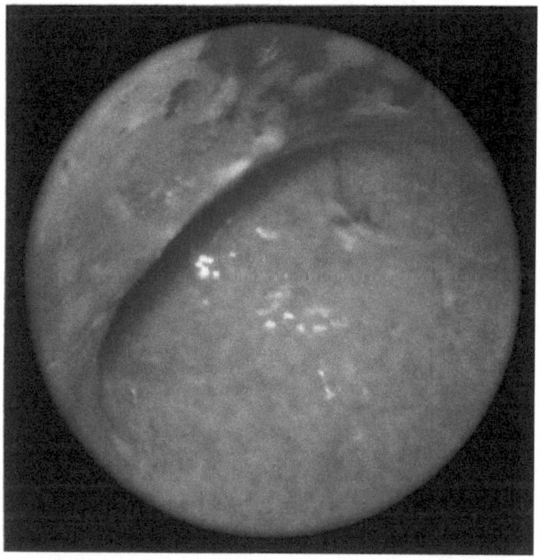
1

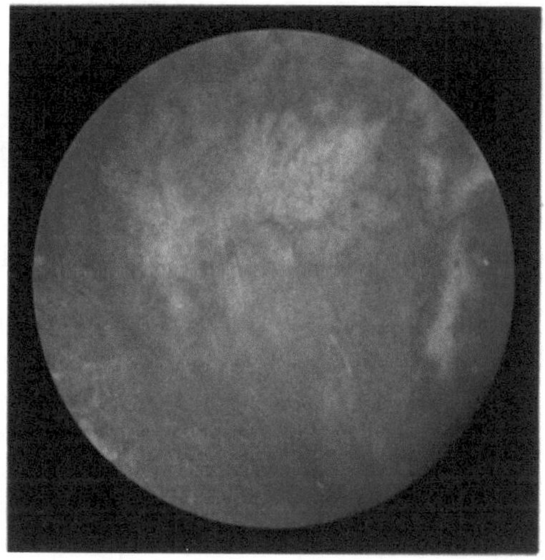
2

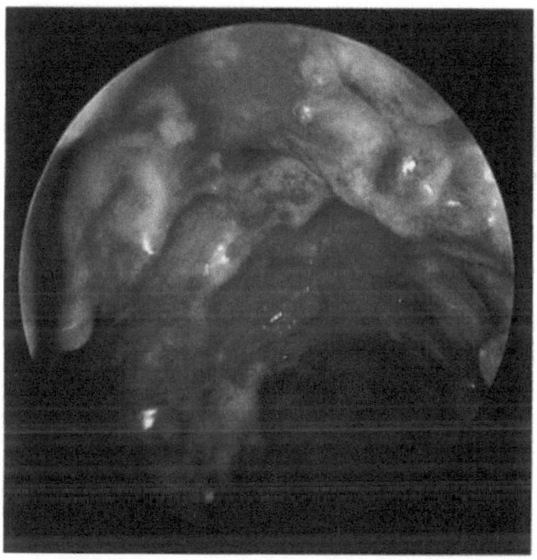
3

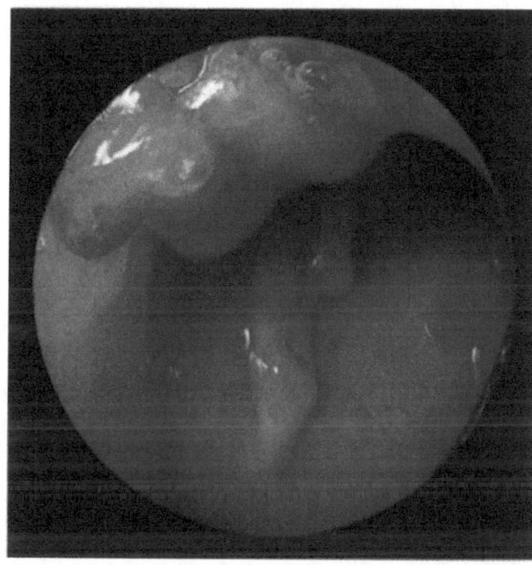
4

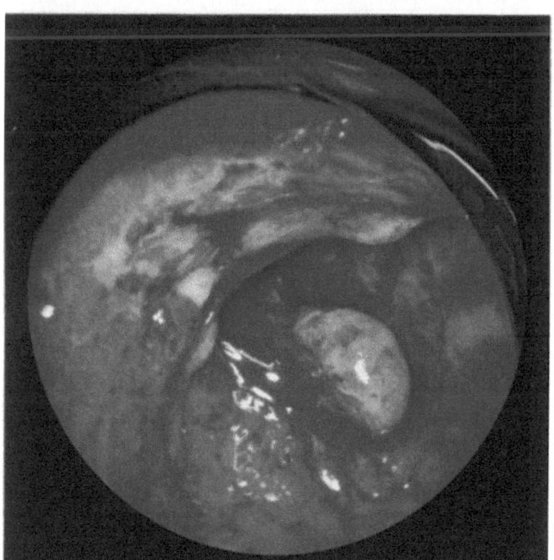
5

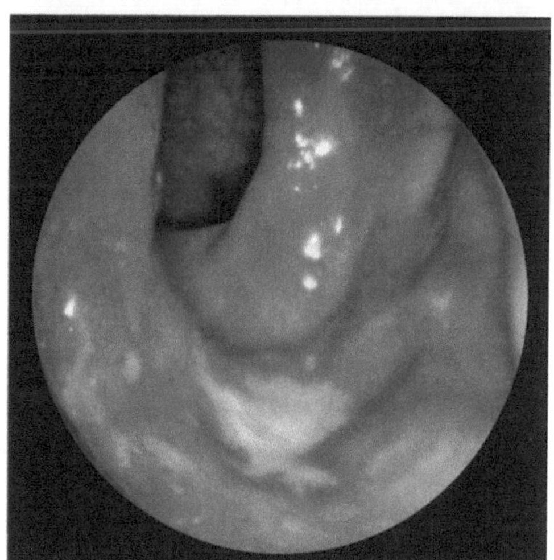
6

Plate XIII/1–6

1 Aphtous-like, circumscribed lesions in an otherwise normal mucosa. These changes can be an early sign of Crohn's disease. They are not demonstrable radiologically. They are not, however, specific for Crohn's disease and can be caused by allergic or bacterially induced inflammatory colitis.

2 Crohn's disease of the rectum. In the normal mucosa, one finds deeply imprinted ulcers in the right side of the bowel wall.

3 Crohn's disease of the rectum (same case as in 2 above). Here we find deep longitudinal ulcers in an otherwise minimally changed rectal mucosa. Clinically there was diarrhea without bleeding. In the biopsy, epitheloid granulomata and Langhans' giant cells were demonstrable.

4 Crohn's disease of the rectum. A close-up view of the ulcerations in the mucosa is presented.

5 Solitary ulcer in Crohn's disease. At the base of a fold, there is a whitish-covered, irregularly appearing ulcer that was the only manifestation of Crohn's disease. The diagnosis was established histologically by biopsy of this area.

6 Fulminant Crohn's disease. In the foreground are two deep ulcers filled with pus. After a latent period of 6 months, during which the only manifestation of the disease had been an anal fistula, a sudden acute reactivation followed with involvement of the whole colon.

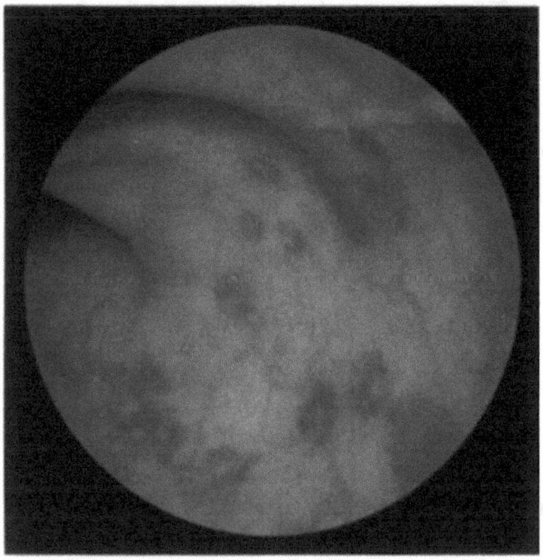

1

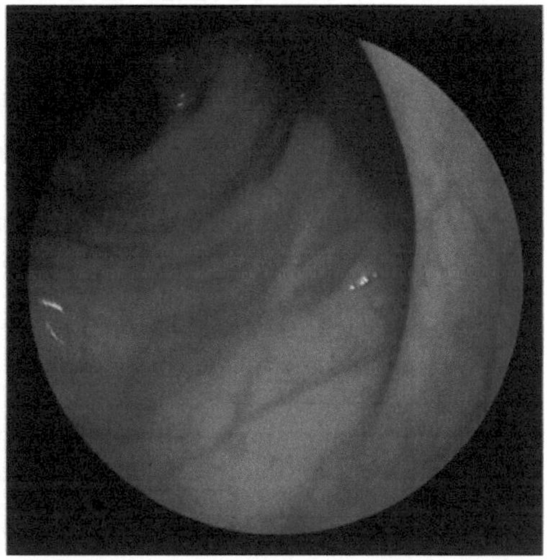

2

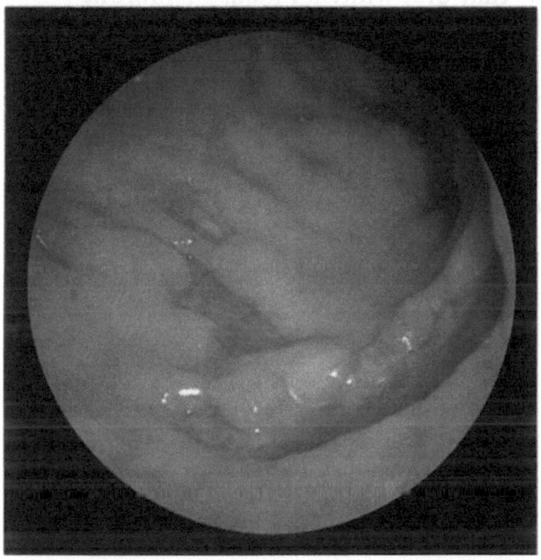

3

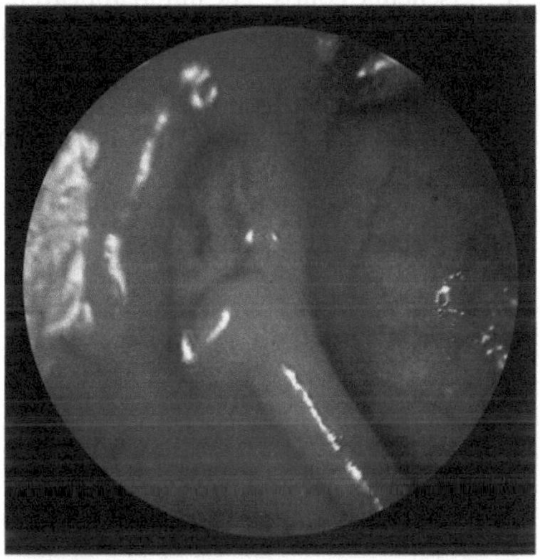

4

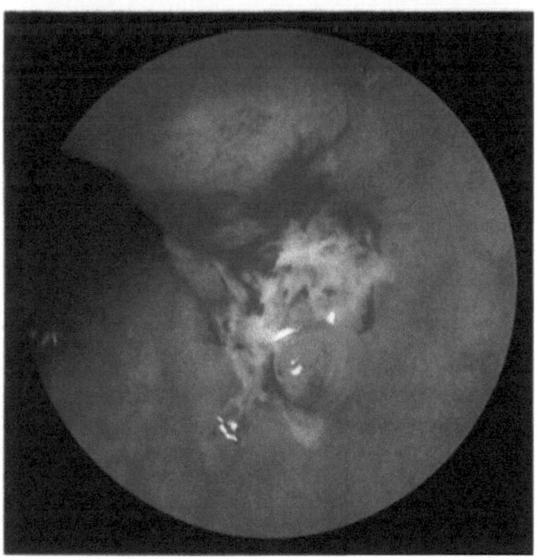

5

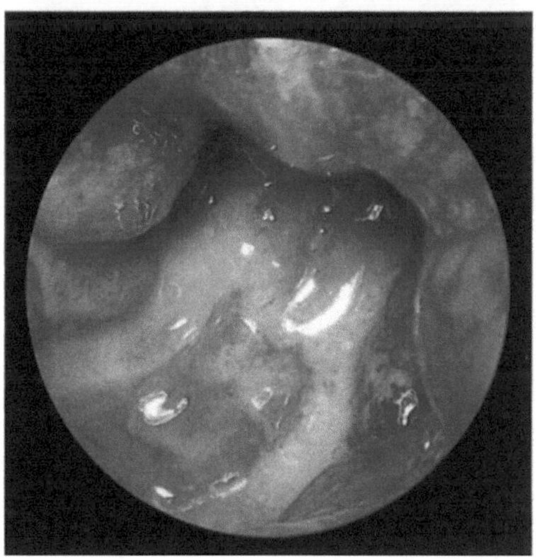

6

Plate XIV/1–6

1 Anastomosis after ileocolostomy in a case of Crohn's disease. In the foreground the anastomotic junction is visible with inflammatory reddening. Subsequently, a stenosis developed in the anastomosis with an extension of the involvement of Crohn's disease to the entire small bowel.

2 Mucosa with a "cobblestone" appearance. In this case, the rectum was spared and the mucosal alterations were only visible on colonoscopy.

3 Pseudomembranous colitis following long-term treatment with orally administered antibiotics. The membrane disappeared after discontinuing the antibiotics. Compare Plate XIV/4, similar picture but different etiology.

4 Ischemic colitis. The initial appearance is that of a whitish mucus membrane with necrosis, later the picture resembles ulcerative colitis.

5 Sigmoid diverticulosis. The view into the diverticular sac is impressive. Diverticula are practically never seen during rectoscopy.

6 Swollen fold. The colon wall is thickened with early stenosis as a consequence of diverticulitis.

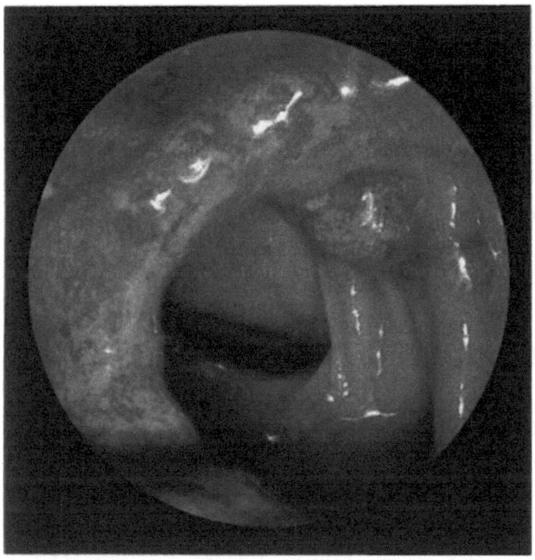

1

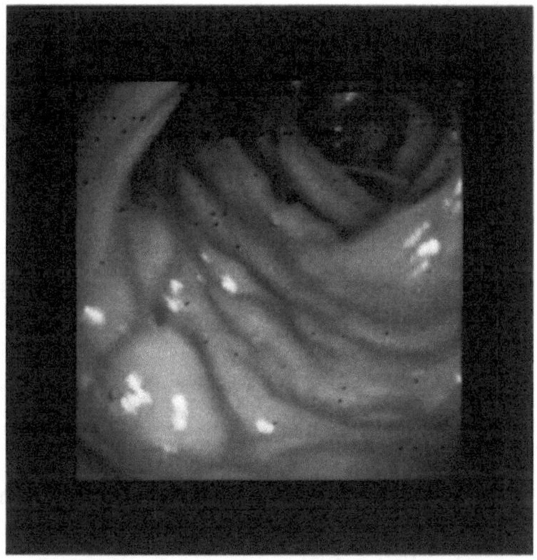

2

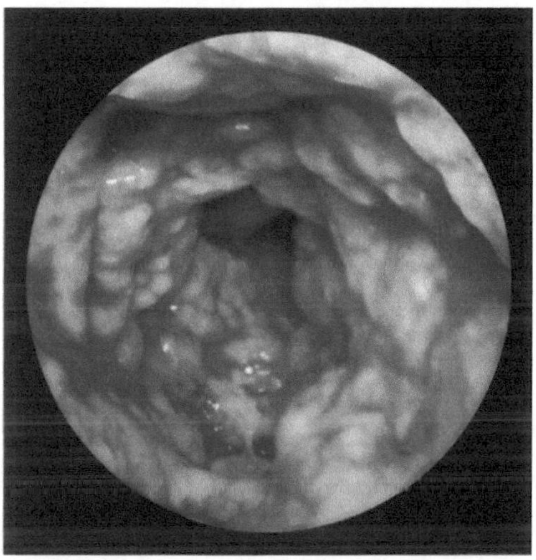

3

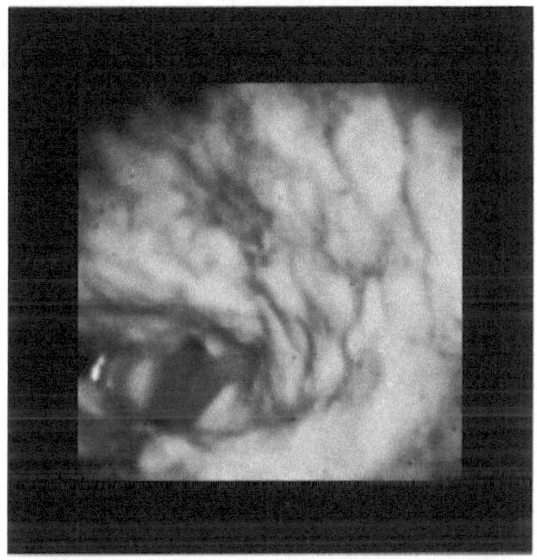

4

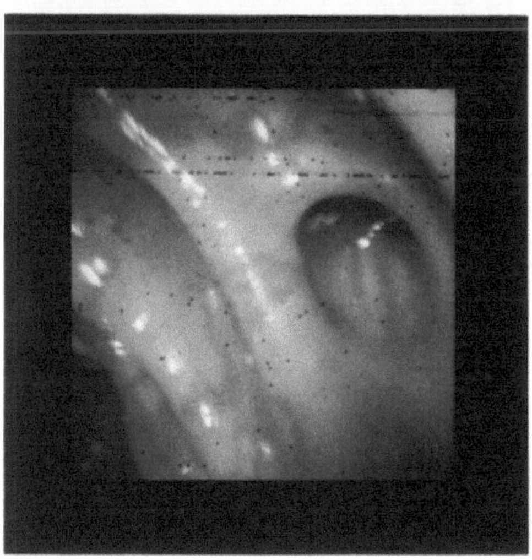

5

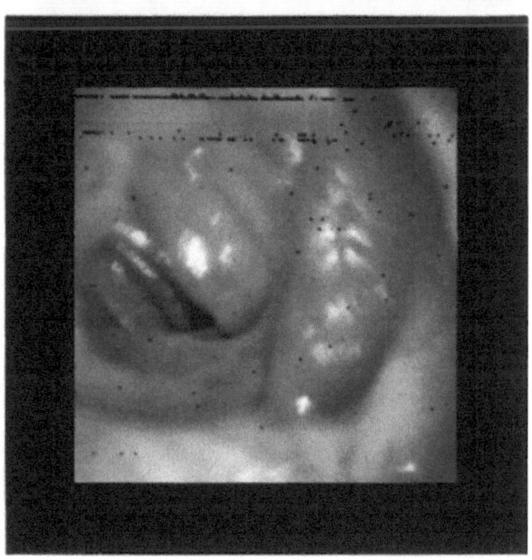

6

Plate XV/1–6

1 Hyperplastic reactive polyp.

2 Papillary adenoma with particularly prominent superficial vascularity.

3 Pedunculated papillary adenoma in the rectum.

4 Condition following electroresection using the high-frequency diathermy loop. A wide necrotic area is apparent at the resection site with sufficient pedicle remaining to give a safety margin to the bowel wall.

5 Broad-based, pea-sized adenoma in the rectum.

6 Condition following electroresection of an adenoma (Plate XV/5). Collar-like necrosis with too deep a resection. The danger of perforation exists. This is tolerable on the posterior wall of the rectum since perforation is not likely in this area.

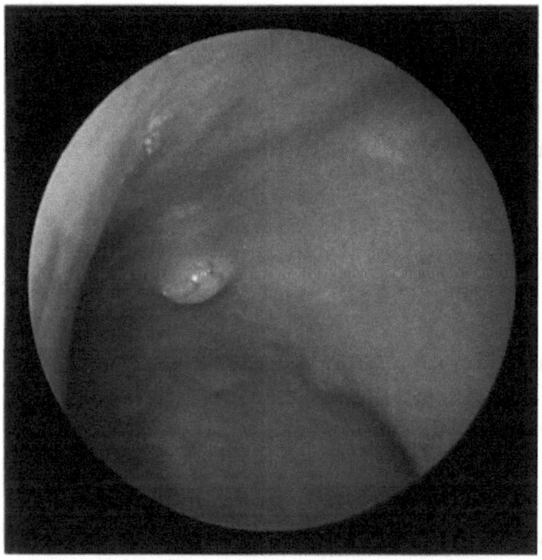
1
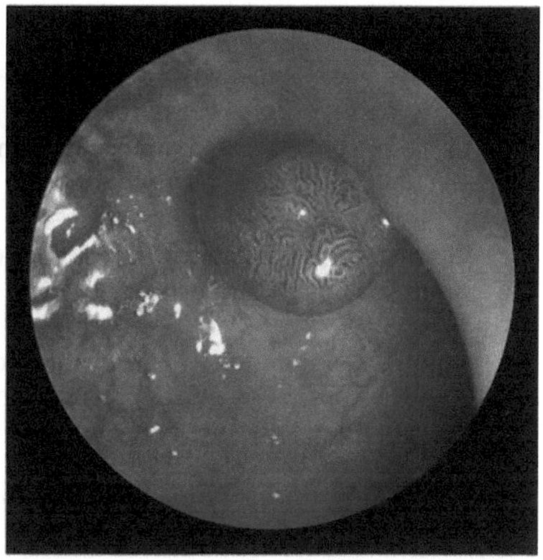
2
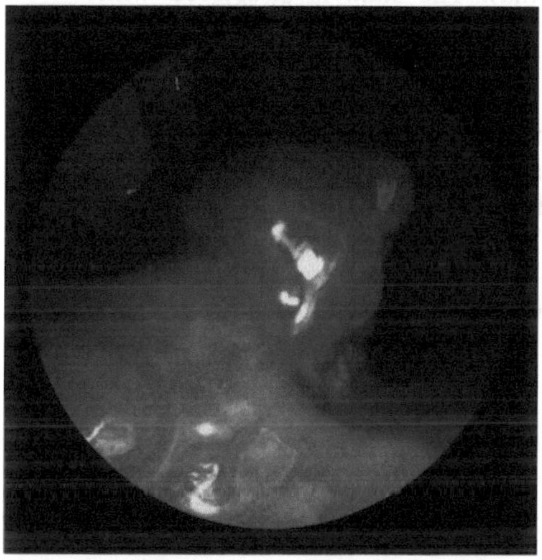
3
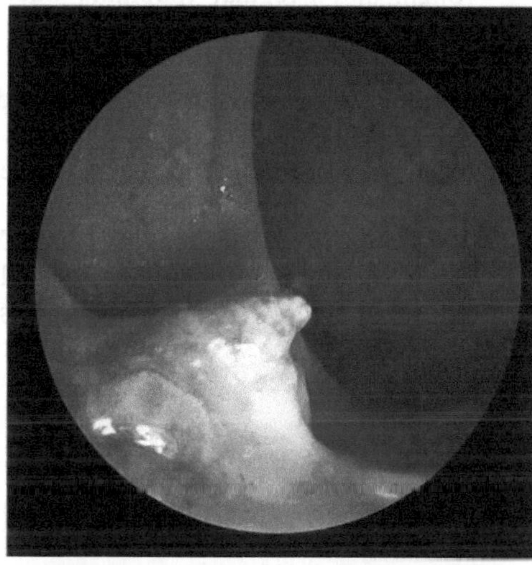
4
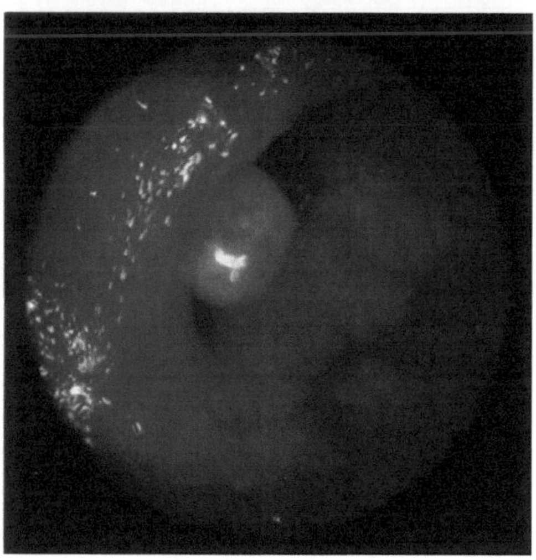
5
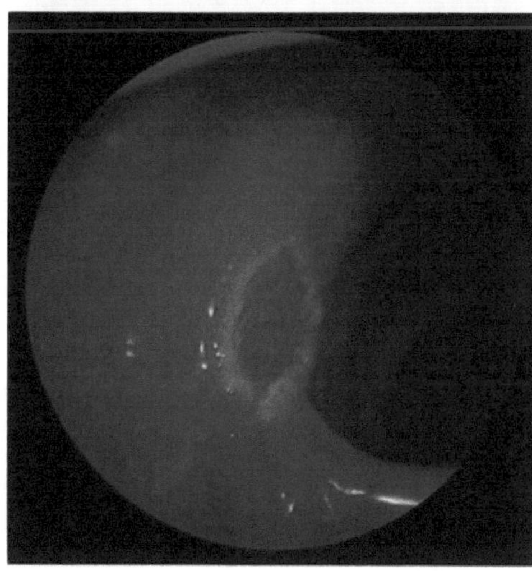
6

Plate XVI/1–6

1 Large pedunculated papillary adenoma in the rectum with focal carcinoma and smooth surface partially covered with stool.

2 Plum-sized pedunculated papillary adenoma with focal carcinoma. Cobblestone-like, irregular surface.

3 Villous adenoma in the rectum. Grass-like arrangement. Upon contact with the forceps, one appreciates a soft, spongy, finger-like, slimy surface. On palpation, the surface feels velvet-like.

4 This pedunculated polyp was resected with the high-frequency diathermy snare from the splenic flexure and was retrieved. The polyp is ragged, rough, and irregular (papillary adenoma). The stalk is discolored white from coagulation.

5/6 Pneumatosis cystoides. A 28-year-old patient who had had blood in the stool 2 years ago. Rectoscopy showed hemorrhoids and the barium contrast X-ray was normal. One year ago there had been increasing gas, a feeling of fullness, and blood with mucus in the stool. Endoscopically, the protrusions appeared to be polyps (Plate XVI/5). During closure of the polyp snare, submucosal air bubbles formed. After resection of the polyp, a cavity remained (Plate XVI/6). The impressive radiologic finding improved after 8 days treatment with oxygen inhalation.

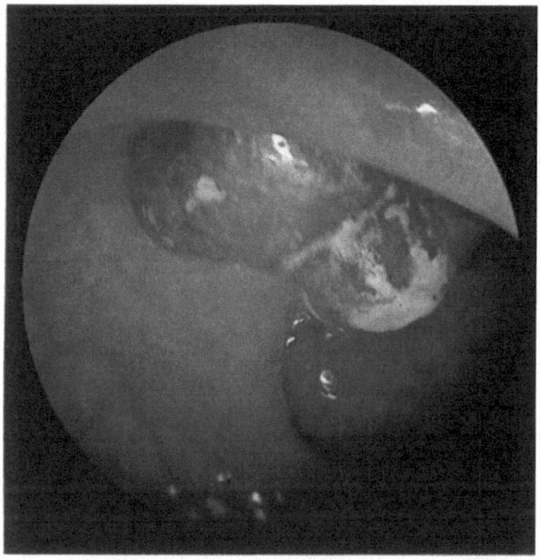
1

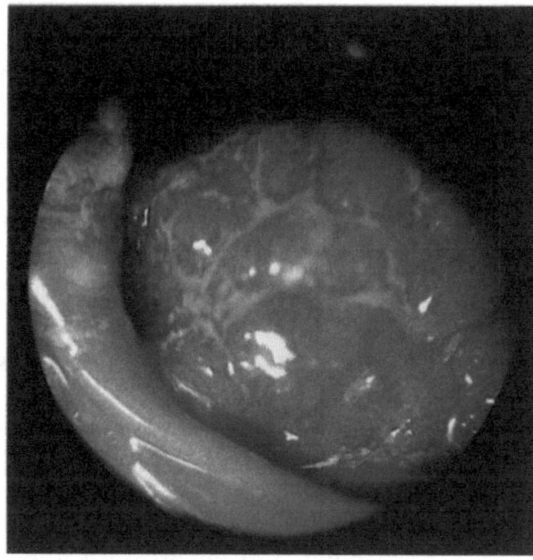
2

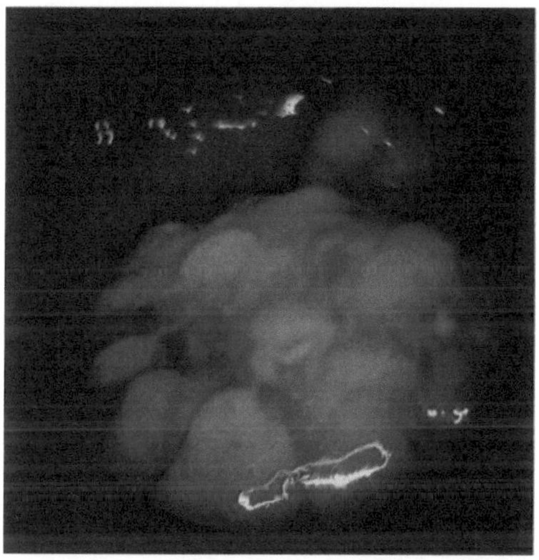
3

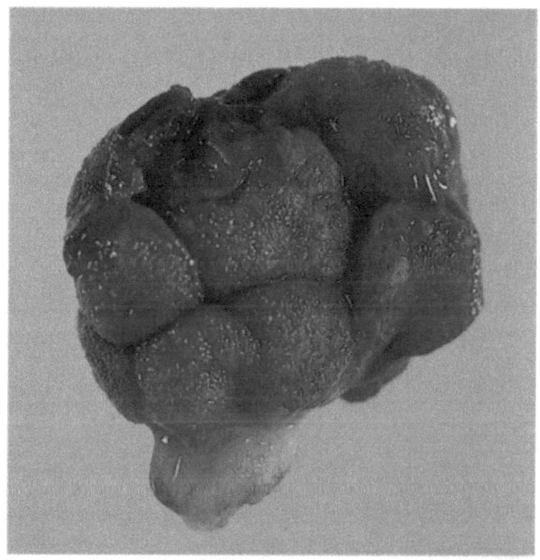
4

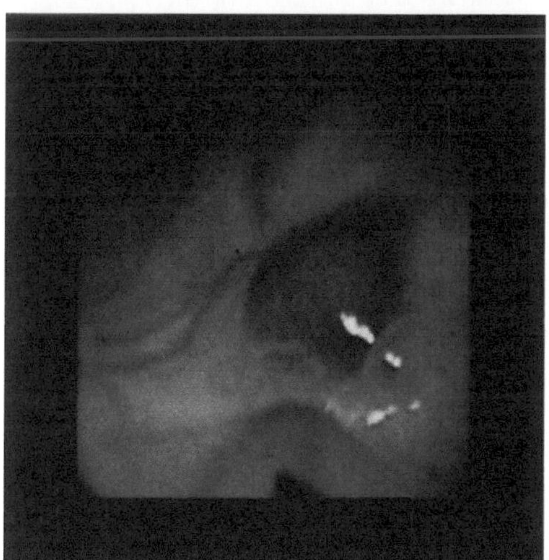
5

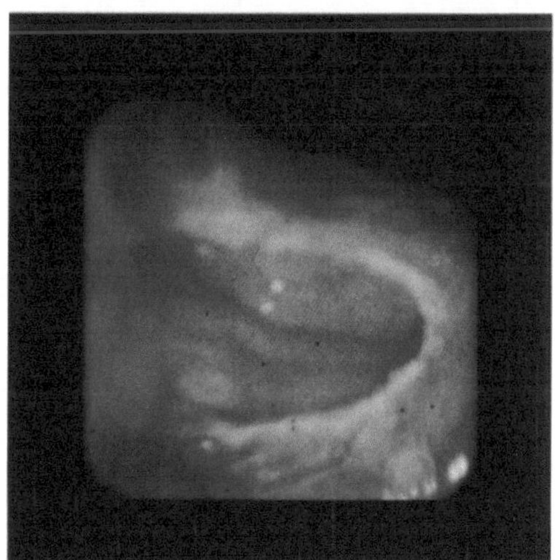
6

Plate XVII/1–6

1 Familial polyposis in the rectum. Multiple papillary adenomas of varying size; partly sessile, partly pedunculated.

2 Malignant polyp in foreground in a case of familial polyposis. In the background several small polyps are visible.

3 Familial polyposis. Closely packed, sessile polyps.

4 Colon resection (Plate XVII/3) showing the rectum.

Peutz-Jeghers Syndrome

5 Typical pigmentation on both upper eyelids and in the base of the nose.

6 Typical Peutz-Jeghers polyp with branch-like configuration.

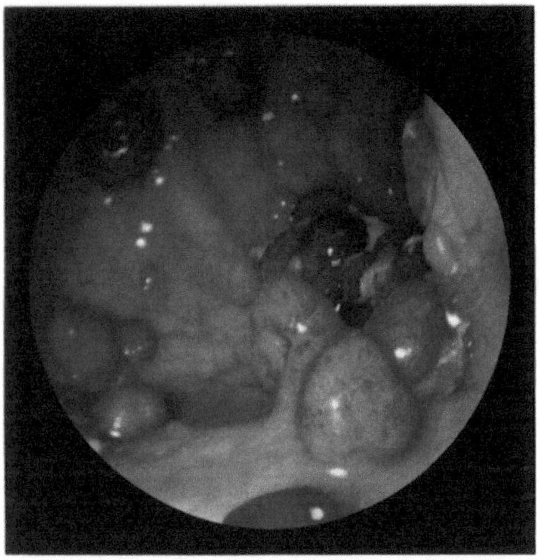
1

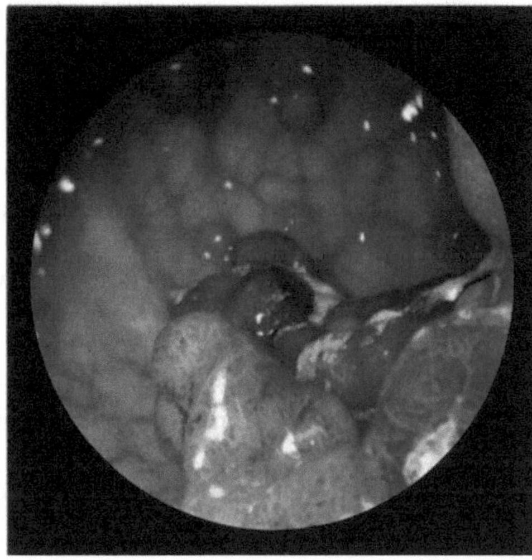
2

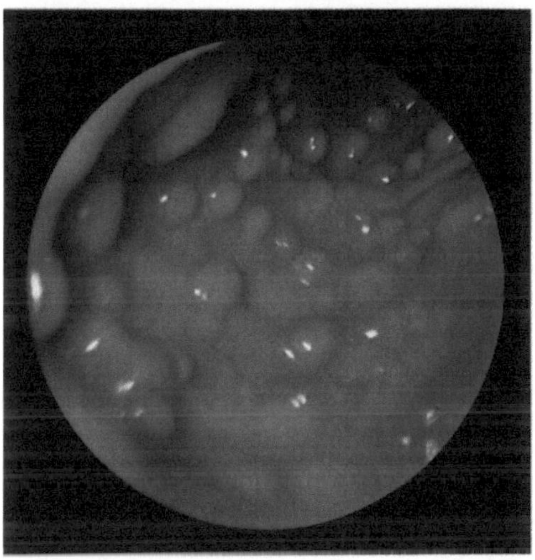
3

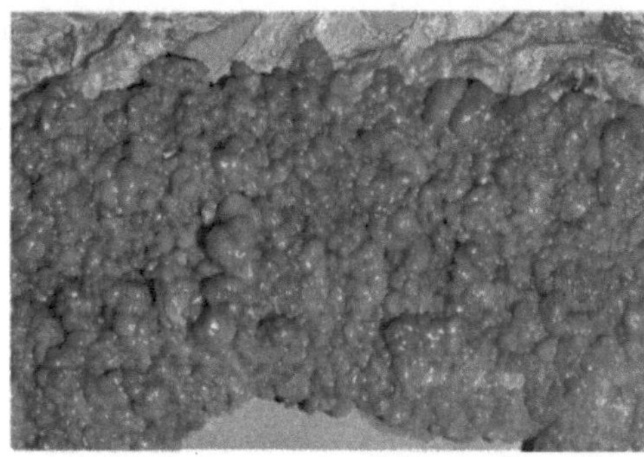
4

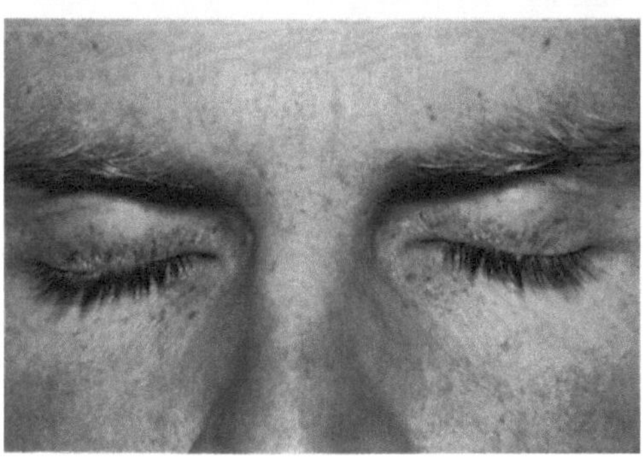
5

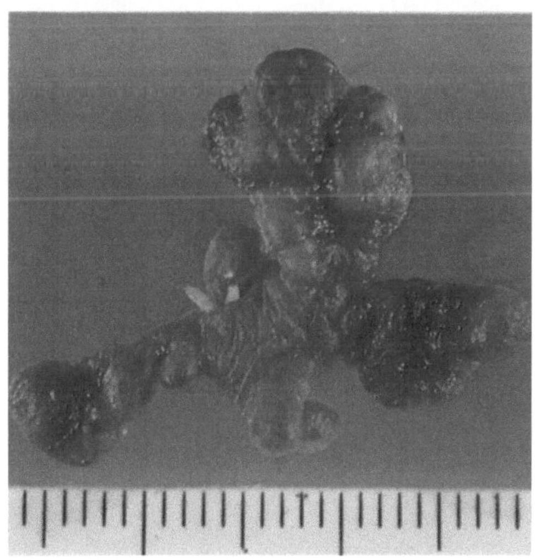
6

Plate XVIII/1–6

1 Polypoid rectal carcinoma with large area of necrosis and obvious bleeding.

2 Circular, stenosing, bleeding rectal carcinoma.

3 Small carcinoma, confined to the wall in the ascending colon that was diagnosed by colonoscopy.

4 Recurrent genital carcinoma that has grown into the rectum. Not grossly distinguishable from a polypoid rectal carcinoma.

5 Infiltration into the rectum in a case of Brill-Symmers disease (giant follicular lymphoblastoma).

6 Leukemic infiltration in the rectum in a case of chronic lymphatic leukemia.

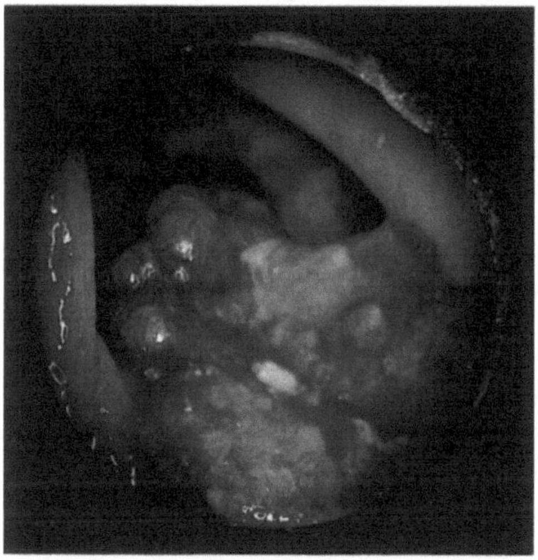
1

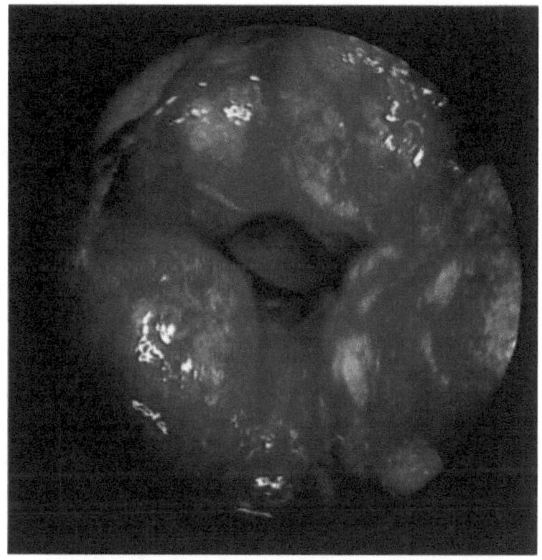
2

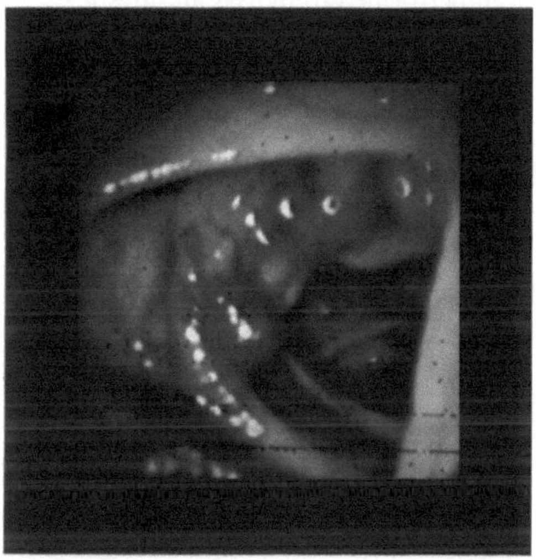
3

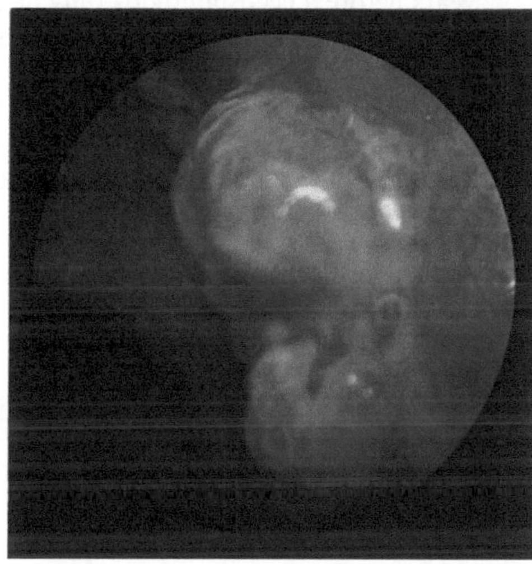
4

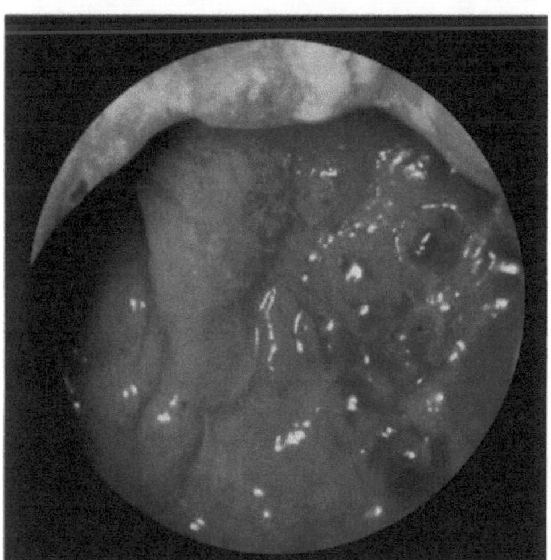
5

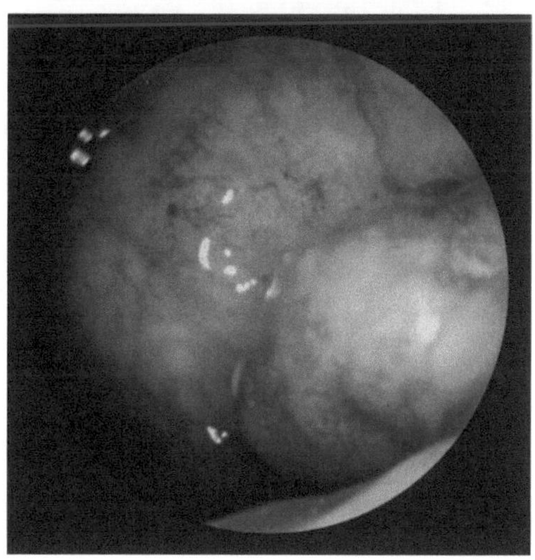
6

Plate XIX/1–6

1 Solitary rectal ulcer. Histologically, the changes were those of inflammation; no evidence of Crohn's disease.

2 Rectovesicular fistula after radiation therapy to a gynecologic carcinoma: Mucopurulent lining with granulation tissue in the anterior rectal wall.

3 As a solitary manifestation of Crohn's disease following ileotransverse colostomy, this rectovaginal fistula remained. Air and stool came out of the vagina. On digital examination, the defect was in close proximity behind the sphincter (lower portion in picture).

4 Cul-de-sac of approximately 6 cm in length, 18 cm above the anus, 27 years before a cecosigmoidostomy had been performed to bypass an intestinal obstruction with subsequent re-establishment of the bowel continuity.

5 Tarry stool in the rectum.

6 Parasite in the rectum (oxyuris, enterobius vermicularis).

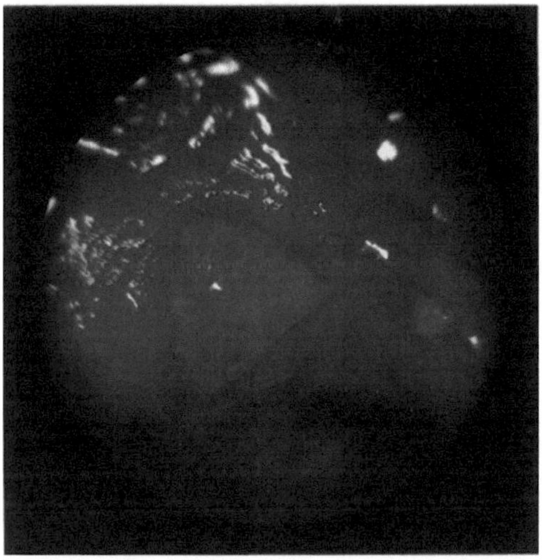
1

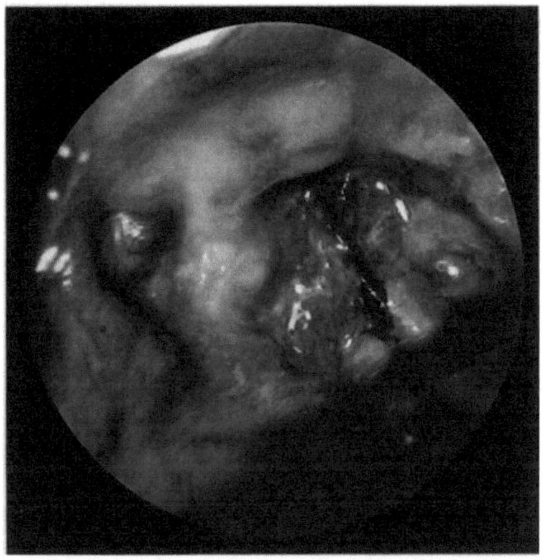
2

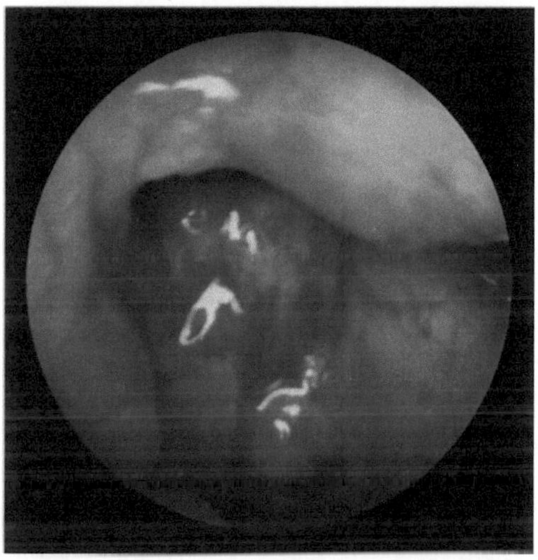
3

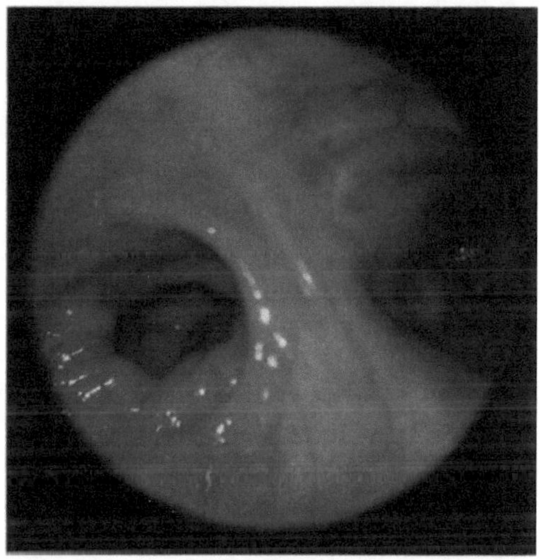
4

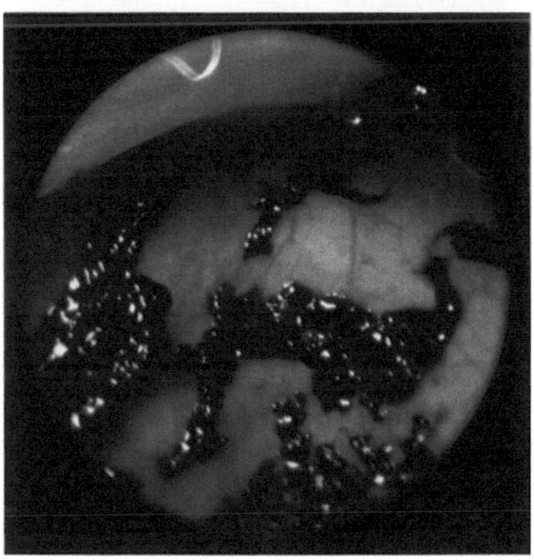
5

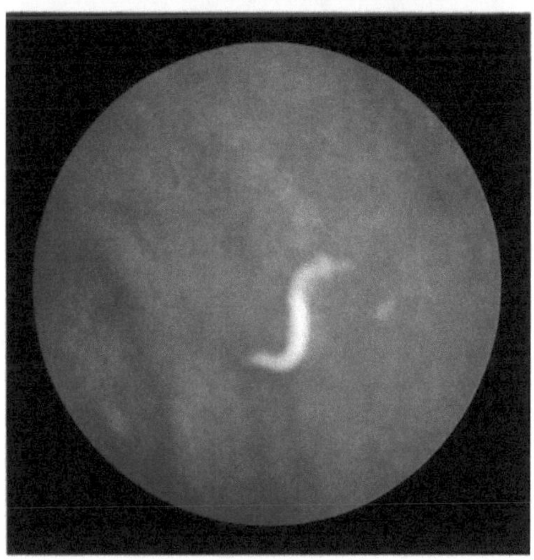
6

Subject Index

MIX
Papier aus verantwortungsvollen Quellen
Paper from responsible sources
FSC® C105338

If you have any concerns about our products,
you can contact us on
ProductSafety@springernature.com

In case Publisher is established outside the EU,
the EU authorized representative is:
Springer Nature Customer Service Center GmbH
Europaplatz 3, 69115 Heidelberg, Germany

Printed by Libri Plureos GmbH
in Hamburg, Germany